ACEP Master Series Courses

ACEP Master Series courses are available to accompany the following texts.

Sport Science

Coaches Guide to Sport Psychology by Rainer Martens discusses motivation, communication, leadership, and how to develop a variety of psychological skills.

Coaches Guide to Sport Physiology by Brian Sharkey leads coaches through the development of fitness-training programs suitable for their athletes.

Coaches Guide to Teaching Sport Skills by Robert Christina and Daniel Corcos uses practical examples to take coaches through the teaching/learning process.

Coaches Guide to Nutrition and Weight Control by Patricia Eisenman, Stephen Johnson, and Joan Benson provides practical guidelines to help coaches assist athletes in losing, gaining, or maintaining weight safely.

Coaches Guide to Social Issues in Sport by Jay Coakley and Robert Hughes examines how age, race, gender, and culture influence sport participation.

Coaches Guide to Sport Biomechanics describes the mechanical principles involved in sport movements.

Sports Medicine

Coaches Guide to Sport Injuries by J. David Bergeron and Holly Wilson Greene gives coaches information on injury prevention, emergency care, and follow-up procedures.

Coaches Guide to Sport Rehabilitation by Steven Tippett explains both the coach's role in rehabilitation and the process of rehabilitation as directed by health-care professionals.

Coaches Guide to Drugs and Sport examines the effects of a variety of abused drugs and the coach's role in combatting drug use.

Sport Management

Coaches Guide to Sport Law by Gary Nygaard and Thomas Boone explains the coach's legal duties in easy-to-understand terms.

Coaches Guide to Time Management by Charles Kozoll explains how to improve organization and avoid time-related stresses.

Coaches Guide to Sport Administration by Larry Leith provides guidelines to help coaches plan, organize, lead, and control their team's success.

Each course consists of a *Coaches Guide, Study Guide*, and *Workbook*. ACEP certification is awarded for successful course completion. For more information, please contact

ACEP
Box 5076
Champaign, IL 61825-5076
1-800-342-5457
1-800-334-3665 (in Illinois)

SECOND EDITION

Coaches Guide to

NUTRITION AND
WEIGHT CONTROL

A publication for the
American Coaching Effectiveness Program
Master Series Sport Science Curriculum

Patricia A. Eisenman, PhD
Stephen C. Johnson, PhD
Joan E. Benson, MS
University of Utah

Leisure Press
Champaign, Illinois

Library of Congress Cataloging-in-Publication Data

Eisenman, Patricia.
  Coaches guide to nutrition and weight control / Patricia A.
Eisenman, Stephen C. Johnson, Joan E. Benson. -- 2nd ed.
    p.   cm.
  Rev. ed. of: Coaches' guide to nutrition & weight control.
  "A publication for the American Coaching Effectiveness Program,
master series sport science curriculum."
  Bibliography: p.
  Includes index.
  ISBN 0-88011-365-0
  1. Athletes--Nutrition. 2. Reducing. I. Johnson, Stephen C.,
1950-   . II. Benson, Joan E., 1954-   . III. Eisenman, Patricia.
Coaches' guide to nutrition & weight control. IV. American Coaching
Effectiveness Program. V. Title.
TX361.A8E4   1990
613.2'5'088796--dc20   89-2204
                                                          CIP

ISBN: 0-88011-365-0

Developmental Editor: Linda Anne Bump, PhD
Copyeditor: Barbara Walsh
Assistant Editor: Julia Anderson
Proofreader: Linda Siegel
Production Director: Ernie Noa
Typesetter: Yvonne Winsor
Text Design: Keith Blomberg
Text Layout: Denise Lowry
Cover Design: Jack W. Davis
Interior Art: Gary Lapelle and Raneé Rogers
Printer: Versa Press

Printed in the United States of America

10 9 8 7 6 5 4 3 2

Leisure Press
A Division of Human Kinetics Publishers, Inc.
Box 5076, Champaign, IL 61825-5076
1-800-747-4457

Contents

Introduction

These are exciting times to be involved in sport. Every year millions of children and adults begin participating in a variety of sports. Although there are numerous reasons why so many are initially attracted to sport, quality coaching is a major factor in why athletes decide to continue. Good coaches make the experience fun, challenging, rewarding, and safe. On the other hand, many athletes can tell horror stories about bad coaches they have had. Coaches who force athletes to practice without water breaks or those who set unrealistic performance weight goals for their athletes are not evil people. It is much more likely that they are unaware of the sport sciences, and therefore lack the knowledge to establish a performance environment that lets athletes have fun while they improve their sport skills and abilities. The purpose of the *Coaches Guide to Nutrition and Weight Control* is to communicate scientific information to coaches so that they can help athletes perform better, enjoy the experience more, and, in the long run, be more successful.

Information from a number of sciences, including nutrition, physiology, and biochemistry, has been incorporated into this book. This material will assist you in learning how to help your athletes optimize their performance potential. This information cannot substitute for your well-planned practices; practice and training sessions are designed to develop skills and conditioning levels, and no magical foods or supplements can replace practice and hard work. But this book presents information you can use to ensure that your athletes do not have to carry excess fat pounds and will have sufficient energy to train hard and go all-out during competitions.

The three parts of the book contain facts and suggestions that will help you manage your athletes' body weight and energy levels. Designed to introduce you to the scientific basis of weight control and sport nutrition, the three sections provide you with some practical strategies for implementing your newly acquired scientific information. A brief examination of each of the three sections should show you how this book can help you become a better coach.

PART I—THE BASICS

The first chapter in this section explains how an understanding of weight control and energy management can influence athletes. Chapter 2 introduces you to the concept that body weight is composed of fat weight and lean weight. This information is critical to understanding weight control for athletes because an athlete's optimal weight means attaining the appropriate balance of lean weight and fat weight. It is more complicated than simply setting a body weight goal. Chapter 2 also discusses a body composition appraisal technique that coaches can implement. Knowledge of the concept of body composition is critical to understanding the strategies for losing fat and gaining lean weight that are presented later in the book.

The first part of the book also presents the basic concept of a balanced diet. Chapter 3 teaches what classes of nutrients are important for a good diet and assists you in acquiring some skills for helping your athletes learn about selecting balanced diets. Chapter 4 builds upon this nutritional knowledge base by providing a more in-depth analysis of two components of a balanced diet—fats and carbohydrates. The chemical composition of fats and carbohydrates, as well as information about good food sources, is presented to give you a better appreciation for the importance of fats and carbohydrates as energy sources for your athletes. Chapter 5 highlights the processes involved in releasing the energy stored in the fuel foods. Knowledge about the energy systems the body uses for various types and intensities of exercise is essential for helping your athletes adopt effective energy-management eating strategies.

PART II— NUTRITIONAL COMPONENTS

The second section of the book elaborates upon the components of a balanced diet introduced in chapter 3. Because fats and carbohydrates were presented earlier to facilitate your understanding of the energy systems, a chapter on amino acids and proteins begins this section. Although these substances are not major fuel foods, they are critical constituents of the athlete's diet. Chapter 6 provides you with a knowledge base for an examination of the merits of the various amino acid and protein supplements that are marketed so heavily to athletes. Numerous commercial products also contain various combinations of vitamins and minerals. The information presented in chapters 7 and 8 should help you understand and communicate to your athletes that eating foods that are rich sources of vitamins and minerals should take priority over expensive supplementation plans.

Chapter 9 focuses on the critical role of water for the performer. In this chapter you will learn that water is an essential component of body weight and that dehydrating techniques for the purpose of losing weight may impair performance. Such techniques can also be hazardous, as noted in the chapter. Chapter 10 examines the role of electrolytes in the optimal functioning of the athlete. In addition to learning about how exercise can disrupt electrolyte balances, you will learn how water and electrolyte replacement strategies go hand in hand.

PART III— USING YOUR KNOWLEDGE

Knowing how to devise safe and effective programs that enable your athletes to work toward optimal performance weights is consistent with good coaching. It is also critical that coaches not allow either weight loss or weight gain strategies to interfere with athletes' health or energy levels.

Chapter 11 provides guidelines for helping athletes set realistic fat loss goals. Information about appropriate eating goals is also presented. Although every effort should be made to provide athletes with sound scientific strategies for losing fat weight, the relatively high incidence of eating disorders, particularly among female athletes, means that coaches need to be aware of the inappropriate strategies that some athletes might adopt to reach their desired body weight. Chapter 12 includes information to sensitize coaches to the problem of eating disorders. This chapter was not designed to prepare coaches to diagnose eating disorders; however, the information should help you recognize the signs and symptoms of inappropriate behaviors and find professional assistance for athletes who may have or may be developing eating disorders.

The issues surrounding gaining lean weight are different from those associated with fat loss, but there are still some potential pitfalls involved. The primary one is that if athletes eat high-fat foods to stimulate weight gain, they may increase body fat levels, blood fat levels, or both. Excessive weight gain may also result in elevated blood pressure for some athletes. Chapter 13 presents material that should help you design weight gain programs that protect your athletes from these potential problems.

Regardless of whether fat loss or additional lean weight is indicated for a given athlete, that athlete needs to have adequate energy to train and to perform. Chapter 14 includes high-performance diet information so that you can help your athletes optimize their energy levels. The principles and ideas presented in this chapter reinforce the need for athletes to eat foods high in carbohydrate and low in fat. The chapter also presents some practical strategies to encourage your athletes to make the transition from the high-fat diet typical of most Americans to the high-carbohydrate diet that is essential for optimal performance, weight control, and health.

The final chapter in this book emphasizes that one of the most effective strategies for motivating athletes to eat appropriately and train regularly is for the coach to serve as a role model. This chapter challenges you to appraise your own body composition and dietary habits. If they are not quite where they should be, use the material in this book to set some reasonable goals and structure some new dietary habits for yourself.

HOW TO USE THIS BOOK

In all the chapters of this book, we have tried to bridge the gap between research and practice by systematically examining both the ''why'' and the ''how'' of nutrition and weight control. We think that the examples presented in this book should help you to see the importance of using nutrition and weight control information on a day-to-day basis as you coach. This book is not the type that you can read once and then put away. We encourage you to review the table of contents and scan the chapters to get a feel for the nature of the material presented. Then reserve some time to systematically read the book chapter by chapter.

Because scientific information is being presented, some of the words used may be new to you. These words have been italicized, and their meaning is explained in the text. At the end of each chapter you will find some specific suggestions for applying the information presented in the chapter. In addition, a *Nutrition and Weight Control Study Guide* is available from the American Coaching Effectiveness Program (ACEP) to facilitate the integration of sport nutrition and weight control into the daily business of coaching athletes. For more information, contact ACEP at

Box 5076
Champaign, IL 61825-5076
1-800-342-5457
1-800-334-3665 (in Illinois)

Once you have read this book, we encourage you to use it as a reference when you need information. In this way, you can assist your athletes to condition themselves for more successful sport participation and to formulate sound nutritional habits. Nothing would make us happier than for this book to help you lead your athletes to success in those endeavors.

PART I
The Basics

Chapter 1
Weight Control and Energy Management

To most Americans, weight control conjures up images of the "Battle of the Bulge"—middle-aged women donning jogging togs and venturing out to the neighborhood health salon, and pot-bellied men exercising to regain the belt size of years gone by. Weight control, for the average person, means watching the numbers drop—or at least not rise—on the bathroom scale.

IDEAL WEIGHT

Weight control in sport, however, means much more than fluctuations on the bathroom scale. To athletes it means striving to achieve the *ideal weight* for optimal performance. Ideal weight is just the right combination of muscle, bone, and fat that gives athletes sufficient size, strength, power, and energy to meet the demands of their sport.

To attain their ideal weight, athletes may need to either lose or gain weight, depending on the particular athlete and sport. Or athletes may be at the proper weight but need to change the proportion of muscle and fat in their bodies. In chapter 2, you will learn how to estimate percent fat, and in subsequent chapters you will learn energy-management procedures you can use to help athletes lose or gain weight safely and effectively. In addition, we will tell you how to feed your athletes with energy-packed, high-octane fuel.

In the competitive world of sport, coaches can no longer afford to use the time-honored binocular scanning method, better known as the "eyeball" technique (see Figure 1.1) for de-

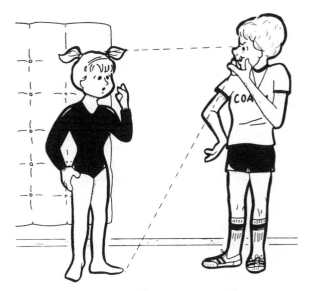

Figure 1.1. The old binocular scanning method, or "eyeball technique," is a poor way to determine the athlete's ideal weight.

termining whether an athlete should lose or gain weight. For that "winning edge," coaches and athletes alike are learning that weight control and nutritional practices to achieve ideal weight must be scientifically managed, just like every other aspect of athletic preparation.

WEIGHT LOSS

Weight control and energy management practices should concern all coaches, not just those in sports that have weight categories or that require tremendous amounts of energy. When athletes are at their ideal weight and are properly fueled, their performance is inevitably better—regardless of the sport being played. Chapters 3, 4, and 5 provide basic information on diet, fuels, and energy systems. Chapters 6 through 10 present the nutritional components required of all healthy diets. The information in these chapters is called upon in chapter 11 to describe safe and effective ways to help athletes lose fat weight.

Let's consider some weight loss examples. As you read each one, consider what you would have done. Then read on and come to understand the healthy approach to weight control.

Football

Earl Edwards and Ken Willard, both professional football players, learned the value of scientifically managed weight control programs (Wilmore & Haskell, 1972). Using body composition procedures developed by sports physiologists, their coaches computed their proportions of muscle and fat. Earl, a defensive lineman, was 20% fat, and Ken, a running back, was 18% fat. When they learned that a defensive lineman's ideal fat weight is 13% to 15% and that a running back's is 6% to 8%, they both altered their eating and exercise habits. Earl dropped to 16% fat and Ken reduced to 11.5% fat.

After losing the fat weight, these men played better than ever, their coaches said. Ken was particularly elated, claiming that not since junior high school had he been able to execute some of the moves he could now.

Baseball

Al Oliver, a baseball player, also benefited from a fat control program (Duda, 1985). In 1981 he had 20% body fat and was a designated hitter with a season batting average of .309. During the off-season, at the suggestion of a conditioning coach, Al lowered his body fat to 12%, which is close to the 10% to 11% ideal for major-league fielders. At this lower fat weight he played outfield and first base for the Montreal Expos and won the 1982 National League batting title with a .331 average.

Distance Running

Tom Fleming, a distance runner, knows that excess fat weight can do more than hinder performance (Costill & Higdon, 1981). In 1978 Tom placed ninth in the Boston Marathon with a time of 2:14:46 despite weighing 169 pounds, which he said was nearly 17 pounds above his normal competitive weight. One thing Tom discovered was that although he still ran well, he recovered much, much more slowly.

Peg Neppel, another distance runner, experienced the effects of utilizing scientific weight management strategies. In her freshman year at Iowa State University, her running times were slower than they had been in high school. At first, Peg didn't know what was wrong, but eventually she realized that the weight she had gained since high school represented unneeded fat. She stepped up her training and eliminated desserts from her diet. As her percent fat decreased, her times improved so much that Peg set a 10,000-meter record for American women.

Gymnastics

Gymnast Nadia Comaneci also experienced the impact of weight fluctuations on her career. In the 1976 Olympics, her optimal body efficiency was reflected in phenomenal performances, but in the months after the Olympics, she grew taller and put on weight. As a result, her performances suffered. Only after a lot of hard work on technique and weight control was Nadia able to regain championship form for the 1980 Olympics.

Wrestling

The athletes just described are only a few of the many athletes who have discovered the importance of proper weight control, but countless others, along with their coaches, still have not. Of all sports, wrestling has the most notorious reputation for poor weight control and energy management practices. Although the abuse is sometimes exaggerated, the bad "rap" is not entirely without foundation, as Davey Samuelson's story illustrates.

When Davey, a high school junior, was faced with the task of losing 19 pounds—from 145 to 126—in 6 days to "make weight" for his Friday wrestling match, he decided to try a new high-fat, high-protein, low-carbohydrate diet he had read about. After 3 days of eating nothing but chicken legs, Davey found himself walking around in a daze, bumping into doors and walls, and daydreaming in school (see Figure 1.2). Practices were a disaster!

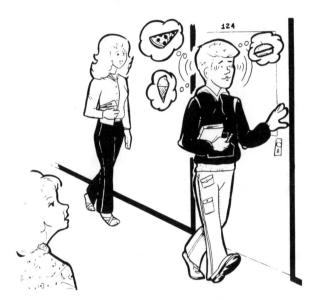

Figure 1.2. High-fat, high-protein, low-carbohydrate diets can leave athletes weak, dazed, and unable to concentrate.

Without his usual energy, he was "hammered" by teammates who seldom beat him, which then brought more criticism from his coach (see Figure 1.3).

Although the diet was working, on Wednesday afternoon Davey still had 7 pounds to lose. So he decided to stop drinking water. By Thursday, he couldn't pass a water fountain without having hallucinations of a giant glass of milk.

Friday morning, a sunken-eyed Davey popped a pill to help him squeeze out even more water. Irritable and depressed, Davey was having trouble getting along at home and at school. He really just wanted to be left alone.

Weigh-in time arrived Friday at 5 P.M. Davey had been in a sauna most of the afternoon, and as he stripped off his clothes, his body resembled a pink prune (see Figure 1.4). He gingerly

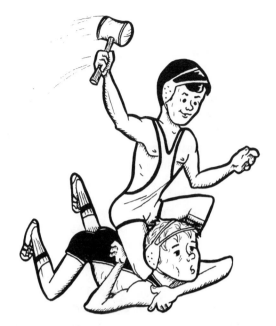

Figure 1.3. Wrestlers who use rapid weight loss techniques frequently find themselves being "hammered" in the waning minutes of practice or a match.

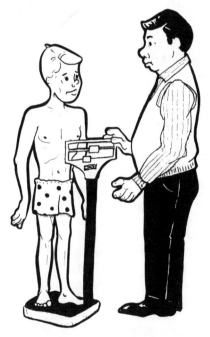

Figure 1.4. Davey need not look so glum; he will "make weight"—this time. But will his shriveled body be able to wrestle?

stepped on the scale, exhaled completely in hopes of shedding air weight, and prayed fervently as the scale's balance bar hovered near the top. The official bent forward for a closer look, then smiled. With the clearance of a gnat's eyelash, Davey had made weight for another week.

Davey leapt from the scale, charged to his locker, gulped down a half gallon of Gatorade, devoured two oranges, and inhaled four chocolate bars. Soon he would be ready to wrestle . . . or so he thought! In actuality, Davey's body was by no means ideally prepared for competition. His performance, as you might imagine, was dismal.

Many wrestlers follow this or similar weight loss procedures week after week, with little regard for how such treatment affects their bodies. In chapter 5 we will explain how energy is made available to the athlete's muscles. In chapter 9 we will examine why the dehydration techniques frequently used by athletes in weight control sports are dangerous and deprive athletes of their peak performance potential.

Volleyball

Stephanie Smith, a member of her collegiate volleyball team, also wanted to lose weight. Her weight problem stemmed from her academic status—the more she worried about staying eligible, the more she ate. As a result of her excessive eating, Stephanie gained weight, and her ability to jump and move on the court deteriorated. Stephanie's coach noticed the weight gain and urged her to lose a few pounds. In desperation, she went on a 3-day fast and severely restricted her water intake. After playing in three vigorous matches on Saturday afternoon, Stephanie became severely dehydrated and was taken to the hospital (see Figure 1.5). She needed to be given intravenous fluids to restore the fluid and fuel balances she had disrupted with her desperate weight control scheme.

In chapters 6 through 10 you will learn about the risk of nutrient deficiencies, dehydration, and electrolyte imbalances that can occur with crash diets. In chapter 11, you will learn how Stephanie should have lost the weight she had gained and still other techniques for helping athletes avoid abusive eating behaviors.

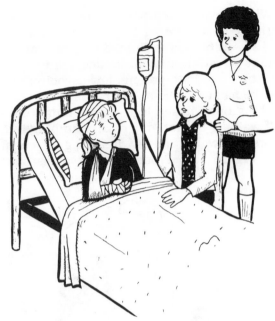

Figure 1.5. Unfortunately, some athletes unknowingly abuse their bodies' water and fuel needs and require medical aid in restoring the appropriate balances.

WEIGHT GAIN

Not all athletes want to lose weight, as Larry Jensen will tell you (see Figure 1.6). After a discouraging football season in which he seldom played, Larry met with his coach to find out what he could do over the summer to improve his chances of playing the following season. He was just too small, his coach explained. Determined to play, Larry went to work. He ate everything in sight, taking special care to pack away lots of eggs, bacon, and red meat, which he thought would build muscle. All summer long, he forced himself to down gigantic milkshakes made with bananas, eggs, nuts, and coconut. He fortified these concoctions with lecithin and other supplements such as wheat germ, zinc, vitamin E, and brewer's yeast.

This gastronomic ordeal helped Larry gain 32 pounds. But when football season arrived, Larry, much to his dismay, did not pass the physical examination. His blood pressure was too high! Most of Larry's gain was fat weight, which probably would not have helped him to play better even if it had not sidelined him

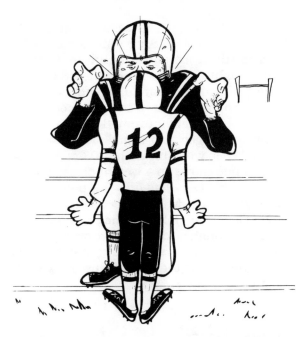

Figure 1.6. Even if opponents tower over your athletes, don't let your players succumb to the temptation of becoming human garbage disposals. Simply being bigger (fatter) will not help them play better!

with high blood pressure. In chapter 13 we will explain how to properly gain muscle weight, *not* fat weight.

SUPPLEMENTATION

Supplementing the diet with various nutrient preparations has become a popular dietary habit. Should you recommend taking supplements? Are they really helpful? Could they actually do harm? These are some of the issues you must consider.

Protein

"Moose" McGraw was a little smarter than Larry Jensen; he knew the difference between muscle weight and fat weight. After a sensational season the previous year, and with rumors surfacing that he would be a contender for the Heisman trophy in the coming season, Moose decided a little more muscle weight would help him be even better.

When the new season began, though, he was hampered by a nagging toe injury. The medical staff thought it was turf toe, but after several weeks it was discovered that Moose had gout—the buildup of excessive uric acid in the blood. He had been consuming so much protein supplement that the uric acid produced by the metabolized protein in his body reached excessive levels. His kidneys were unable to remove all the uric acid, and a very sore toe was the result.

Moose's bout with gout is an example of the "more is better" myth that traps athletes seeking to build their bodies with protein supplements. In chapter 6, you will learn why athletes need not and should not consume excessive quantities of protein.

Iron

For some athletes, however, supplements and extra vitamins may be essential. Ellen Rose, who had been running distance races for 10 years, was feeling tired all the time. Her workouts became a struggle, and her racing times were way below her personal records. She tried to be health-conscious and therefore planned her meals around a high-carbohydrate, low-fat, primarily vegetarian diet. She restricted her intake of salt, refined sugar, white flour, processed foods, additives, red meats, fats, and cholesterol. When Ellen underwent a computerized analysis of her diet, she found that her intake of the major nutrients was adequate, except for iron and zinc. Also, the analysis indicated a routine of high caffeine intake due to her consumption of coffee and diet cola. After consulting with a physician to rule out medical problems and to have blood tests to determine iron levels, Ellen consulted with a sport dietician. Based on blood tests that verified low iron levels, Ellen began daily iron (250 milligrams of ferrous sulfate) and zinc (25 milligrams) supplementation. Within 10 days she noticed an improvement in her running performance. Not only did she feel better, but people began to tell her that she looked better and had more color in her face. Ellen plans to prevent a recurrence of the situation by having her iron status monitored three times a year so that she can alter her diet and supplement intake if necessary. Chapters 7 and 8 will provide you with additional information about how vitamin and mineral needs may be scientifically managed.

THE COACH'S DILEMMA

Most coaches acknowledge the importance of weight control and nutrition for good athletic performance, but many candidly admit that they actually do very little to directly assist their athletes in this area. Why?

Perhaps coaches find it difficult to wade through the quagmire of nutritional and weight control literature that appears in newspapers, on television, and in countless magazines and books. With all the fad diets and "miracle" potions on the market, separating fact from fiction is no easy task. Coaches also may wonder whether weight control methods intended for middle-aged adults are appropriate for young athletes whose bodies demand lots of energy. Or perhaps coaches are more familiar with the traditions of their sports than with the research findings of sport scientists. For example, do you still follow such practices as

- providing the supposedly high-energy steak-and-egg meal before each big game;
- requiring athletes to take salt tablets on hot days;
- using candy bars for quick energy;
- providing expensive fluid replacement formulas thought to be superior to water;
- forbidding athletes to drink cold water; or
- suggesting protein pills as dietary supplements?

Are these really the best practices? Can you tell fact from fiction in the weight control and energy management techniques you use with your athletes?

THE INFORMED COACH

Coach John Stringer can. Bill Ferguson weighed 150 pounds when he reported for wrestling after completing a successful football season. Coach Stringer computed Bill's percent fat using procedures described in chapter 2: It was 14%. Knowing that the ideal percent fat is 5% to 7% for a champion wrestler (American College of Sports Medicine, 1976), Coach Stringer explained to Bill that his *optimal* weight class would be the 137-pound category. Through a carefully planned weight control program supervised by his coach, Bill slowly lost the weight over a 3-month period.

Coach Stringer also urged Gary Landers, who had been wrestling at the 103-pound classification, to move up a weight class by gaining 7 pounds. Gary had only 3% body fat and was just too weak to compete at the lower weight class. Gary followed the coach's advice, and even though he did not have a spectacular season in terms of winning, he enjoyed wrestling more than in the past because he was not constantly hungry.

SUMMARY

The knowledge Coach Stringer used with his athletes is found in the following chapters of this book. We will show you how to determine the ideal weight range for each of your athletes and give you the information you need to help your athletes adjust their weight safely and properly to achieve the right proportion of bone, muscle, and fat. We will explain how to meet the nutritional needs not of sedentary middle-aged adults but of high-energy-consuming athletes. And we will dispel many nutritional myths that abound in sport.

In subsequent chapters, you will learn the following:

1. How muscles release energy
2. Which foods best fuel these energy-releasing processes
3. How proteins and amino acids are used by athletes
4. When vitamins and other supplements are needed
5. What vital role water plays in athletic performance
6. Whether electrolytes are also needed
7. Whether high-energy, super-fuel carbohydrate diets are effective

In short, we will present weight control and energy management practices that are based not on opinion or current nutritional fads, but on scientifically proven facts. We challenge you to put them to use in your program.

Chapter 2
Appraising and Monitoring Body Composition

In the last chapter we discussed the importance of ideal weight. Now let's learn more about it and find out how to determine ideal weight ranges by assessing body composition.

Ideal weight is highly individualized. It is weight that allows an athlete to function optimally in his or her chosen sport. *There is no one ideal body weight for all athletes.* An ideal weight for one athlete may be completely inappropriate for another.

THE FACTS ABOUT IDEAL WEIGHT

Helping athletes achieve their ideal weight is more complicated than simply manipulating the numbers that appear when they step on the scale. For example, gymnasts should not only minimize their body weight but should also maximize their strength-to-weight ratio to enhance skill and prevent injuries. Similarly, wrestlers should compete at the weight class in which their strength, endurance, and skill are optimal. Achieving these objectives depends upon understanding three basic facts:

Ideal Weight Facts

Fact 1: The body's weight is composed of many different constituents.

Fact 2: Not all of the body's compartments contribute equally to the body's weight.

Fact 3: Not all of the body's constituents contribute equally to sport performance potential.

Weight Composed of Different Constituents

Muscle tissue, nerve tissue, bones, ligaments, tendons, skin, minerals, and fat are all part of the body's composition (see Figure 2.1). Due to the limitations of their instruments, sport scientists have consolidated these constituents into major component parts. One sophisticated model assumes that there are four component parts to body weight: fat, fat-free water, fat-free mineral, and fat-free protein. Because of the difficulty in measuring each of these compartments, a two-compartment-model approach to body composition is much more prevalent. With this model the two components are lean (or muscle) and fat, as Figure 2.2 shows. This means that body weight is

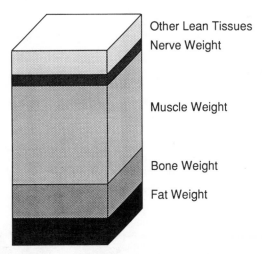

Other Lean Tissues
Nerve Weight

Muscle Weight

Bone Weight

Fat Weight

Figure 2.1. Muscle tissue, nerve tissue, bones, ligaments, tendons, skin, minerals, and fat are all components of body weight.

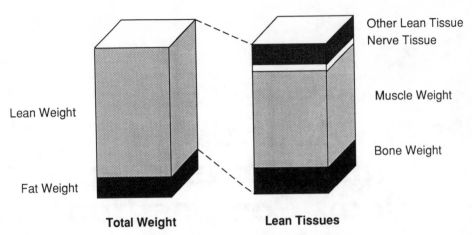

Figure 2.2.   Because of the difficulty in measuring each of the components of body weight, a method has been devised to divide body weight into two compartments: lean weight and fat weight.

assumed to be composed of just lean (or fat-free) weight and fat weight.

Compartments Contribute Unequally to Weight

Fat is less dense than muscle. *Density* refers to the mass of a substance relative to its volume. To illustrate this idea, imagine a balance scale with a one-pound lead pellet on one of the trays. The container with the one-pound lead pellet would not need to be very large (see Figure 2.3). Now imagine you balanced the lead pellet with a pound of feathers; it would take a very large container to hold them. The reason for this disparity in

the size of the containers is due to the difference in the density of lead and of feathers. Lead is quite dense; it has a relatively small volume relative to its weight. Feathers, on the other hand, are not dense; they have a large volume relative to their weight.

The body's lean weight and fat weight also vary in density. Muscle is more dense than fat, and bone is typically more dense than muscle. (In chapter 11 we will discuss situations where dieting and training practices may decrease an athlete's bone density.) Because of the differences in the density of muscle and fat, it is possible that two individuals could have the same height and weight but completely different body dimensions, such as the two girls pictured in Figure 2.4. The girl on the right has 30% fat weight and obviously larger dimen-

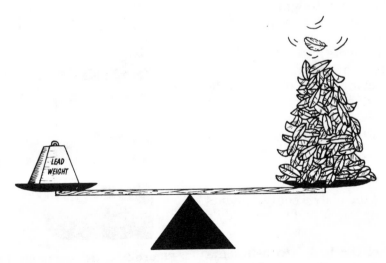

Figure 2.3.   Lead is more dense than feathers, so a pound of feathers takes up more space than a pound of lead.

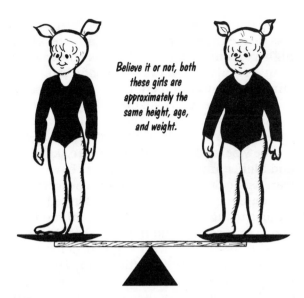

Believe it or not, both these girls are approximately the same height, age, and weight.

Figure 2.4. Fat tissue and lean tissue vary in density, so simply looking at scale weight can be misleading.

sions than the girl on the left, who has only 20% fat.

If the girl on the left is older and her skeleton more mature, this could also contribute to her lower percent fat. The body composition prediction techniques presented in this chapter take age into consideration as a way of calculating the influence of skeletal maturity. After reading this material on density, it should be obvious that ideal weight cannot be determined simply by using scales to weigh athletes.

Constituents Contribute Unequally to Performance Potential

The contraction of the various muscles used to propel the body and enable an athlete to handle such implements as racquets and balls depends on the muscles receiving guiding signals from the nervous system. The nervous system also regulates the work of the heart to pump blood to the muscles, which is fundamental to the execution of sport activities. Without strong bones, the contractile forces of the skeletal muscles could not be used for throwing, running, and jumping. Because the nerves, skeletal muscles, heart, blood vessels, and bones are all part of the body's lean weight, it is readily apparent that lean tissues

are essential to the performance of physical activities.

On the other hand, a large quantity of body fat does not help performance. For example, in a study of 835 high school wrestlers by Tcheng and Tipton (1973), average body fat was 8%, but the 224 wrestlers who had reached the state finals had body fat contents ranging from 4% to 6%. Obviously, the better or more successful wrestlers were also leaner. At this point you should also note that the absolute amount (number of pounds) of lean weight as well as the optimal percent fat varies between sports. Contact sports like football favor high absolute quantities of lean weight, while sports like distance running favor smaller absolute lean weights as well as lower percent fat values (Sinning et al., 1985).

BODY COMPOSITION APPRAISAL

To implement a scientifically managed weight control program, you need some means for determining the athlete's body composition. In other words, you need to find out what percentage of the athlete's body weight is fat weight and what percentage is lean tissue. Such information allows you to know if the athlete has excess fat or needs to gain additional lean weight. Although a number of things need to be considered and a margin of error exists, you can learn to compute your athletes' body composition.

The most accurate procedures for determining body composition, particularly in children, utilize a four-compartment model in which body weight is divided into fat, fat-free water, fat-free mineral, and fat-free protein (Boileau, Lohman, & Slaughter, 1985). Measurement of fat-free mineral and fat-free water content takes the chemical maturity of the youngster into account so that the fat percentages of younger children, who have less mature skeletons and more body water, will not be overestimated. Unfortunately, these procedures are not feasible for the coach's use. Therefore, more practical procedures utilizing a two-compartment model of body composition have been developed, based on what scientists have learned with the more sophisticated four-compartment models.

Hydrostatic Weighing

One of the more accurate two-compartment model techniques for appraising body composition is called *hydrostatic weighing*. With this procedure, an athlete is submerged in water to obtain the underwater weight (see Figure 2.5). When the underwater and the land weights are obtained, a series of calculations

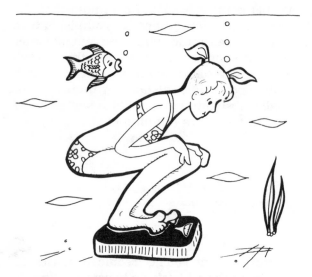

Figure 2.5. Underwater weighing is more than just placing a scale underwater; it is a scientific way of using land weight and underwater weight to calculate body density.

are computed to determine body density. Percent fat may be predicted once body density is determined.

The measurement of underwater weight permits the calculation of body composition because fat and lean tissue do not have the same density. More specifically, fat tissue is less dense than lean tissue. An athlete with a high percent of fat weighs less underwater than an athlete with the same body weight on land but a lower percent of fat. For the same reason, people with a lot of fat float more easily than lean people do. The fat is buoyant because it is less dense than water.

Likewise, children with immature skeletons and higher amounts of body water have lower lean tissue density than adults. The formulas presented in Table 2.1 were derived from studies using the four-compartment model of body composition and indicate that the body density associated with a given percent fat varies with age and sex (Lohman, 1986). By using these formulas, body fat percentages may be predicted by using the body density values obtained from hydrostatic weighing.

Despite its accuracy, underwater weighing is not widely used because the necessary equipment is costly, the procedure requires experienced technicians, and it takes a considerable amount of time. Scientists have, therefore, developed more practical techniques for physicians and coaches to use.

Skinfold Method

Skinfold procedures, or "pinch tests" as they are sometimes called, are much more practical for coaches. These procedures entail measuring the distance across a fold of skin (see Figures 2.6 and 2.7). When you pinch a fold of skin, you also pick up the fat lying under the skin (known as subcutaneous fat). Scientists have observed a relationship be-

Table 2.1
Conversion of Body Density to Percent Fat

Age	Males	Females
13-15	$[(5.07/D^a) - 4.63] \times 100$	$[(5.12/D) - 4.69] \times 100$
15-17	$[(5.03/D) - 4.59] \times 100$	$[(5.07/D) - 4.64] \times 100$
17-20	$[(4.98/D) - 4.53] \times 100$	$[(5.05/D) - 4.61] \times 100$
Over 20	$[(4.95/D) - 4.45] \times 100$	$[(5.03/D) - 4.59] \times 100$

Note. Derived from Lohman (1986).

[a]D = Body density calculated from hydrostatic weighing.

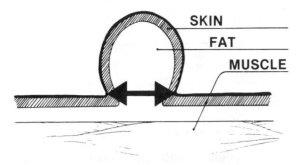

Figure 2.6. Skinfold calipers are used to measure the thickness of the subcutaneous fat in a "pinch" of skin.

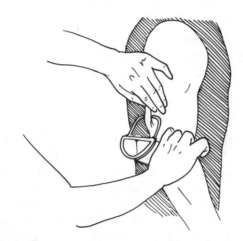

Figure 2.7. The triceps skinfold.

tween the amount of fat stored at selected skinfold sites and the body's total fat. This knowledge is used to predict body composition.

Although the skinfold method is a relatively simple idea, its application does require skill and knowledge. One of the major difficulties with the method is that a number of factors seem to influence where each person deposits subcutaneous fat. Recent research even shows that different types of athletes deposit fat differently. Another problem with the skinfold technique stems from the fact that children and older adults, particularly women, have lower bone densities than young adult males. Consequently, the relationship between subcutaneous fat thickness and body density varies among different populations. Such variability means that different skinfold sites and different prediction equations must be used according to the age, sex, and sport of the specific athlete.

In addition to skinfold procedures, anthropometrical measurements have also been used to predict body composition. The word *anthropometric* refers to the measurement of human beings; anthropometrical techniques involve measuring the circumference of limbs or the trunk (for example, biceps girth and abdominal girth) and measurements of skeletal diameters (for example, ankle width and knee width). The use of such measurements in the prediction of body composition capitalizes on the relationships between skeletal size and the total amount of lean tissue in the body.

Specific procedures for predicting percent fat values of young male and female athletes by using the fat calipers method are fully described in this chapter. You may also want to view Lohman's (1987) video for additional assistance. This method is the more general and hence more useful one for most coaches. Procedures for predicting the fat percentages of adults are presented in chapter 15. In addition, some techniques for using skinfold values to track weight management procedures are presented in the final sections of this chapter.

IMPLEMENTING THE SKINFOLD METHOD

Although the skinfold method has been proven valid, it is not fail-safe. The skill of the person taking the measurements greatly determines its validity. Using fat calipers is a motor skill just like shooting free throws in basketball or driving tee shots in golf. An untrained beginner is less accurate than a well-coached, experienced veteran. So, we will coach you in the proper use of the calipers and then urge you to practice by taking as many measurements as you can.

Obtain Calipers

The first thing you need to do, obviously, is acquire a pair of fat calipers. The sources for purchasing calipers and the approximate costs of the different models are listed on page 14.

The quality of the calipers you purchase is important. If you use less expensive calipers, accuracy and consistency will suffer somewhat. However, a little practice can help improve this accuracy (Hawkins, 1983; Morrow, Fridye, & Monaghen, 1986), and instructions

Sources for Calipers

Product	Vendor
Harpenden skinfold calipers ($250)	Quinton Instruments 2121 Terry Ave. Seattle, WA 98121
Lange skinfold calipers ($150)	Cambridge Scientific Industries 527 Poplar St. Cambridge, MD 21613
Fat-o-meter ($20)	Health and Education Services 2442 Irving Park Rd. Chicago, IL 60618
Adipometer ($5)	Ross Laboratories 625 Cleveland Ave. Columbus, OH 43216

for using one model of calipers are presented in Appendix A. An excellent videotape that presents the calipers technique (*Measuring Body Fat Using Skinfolds*, Lohman, 1987) may be purchased along with a software package to estimate body fat from Human Kinetics, Box 5076, Champaign, IL 61825-5076.

We also must point out that the equations used to compute body composition are based on averages compiled from many individuals. It is possible, therefore, that a given athlete's body build, sex, race, or level of physical maturity might render the equation not entirely accurate for him or her. Even under the best of circumstances, there is as much as a 3% to 5% error in the predictive equations (Lohman, 1981). We mention this margin of error not to discourage your use of this method, but to emphasize that common sense and good judgment must accompany your use of the calipers and calculator. Indeed, we strongly urge that you use calipers rather than the less accurate eyeball method.

Emphasize Composition, Not Absolute Weight

Using the calipers technique helps to emphasize that if athletes have an excess of fat weight, that fat weight should be lost. By appraising body composition, the coach can re-

inforce the concept that just losing weight via dehydration and crash dieting does not enhance athletes' performance potential. Losing fat weight helps. Although we discuss a formula for predicting ideal weight, the calculated values are just a starting point and an educational tool for the athlete. The emphasis should be on adopting appropriate eating and training strategies, not just achieving the calculated ideal weight. This topic is discussed in more detail in chapters 11 and 13.

Select a Skinfold Prediction Formula

Many different formulas have been developed for using skin calipers. The specific formula and the associated skinfolds described here are well documented, relatively simple, and appropriate for young athletes. You are required to take two of the following three skinfold measurements: either the triceps and calf skinfolds or the triceps and subscapular skinfolds.

Each of these measurements is to be taken on the right side of the body on all athletes. You must take considerable care in locating the precise site for the measurement; the accuracy of the test depends on it. Although the following skinfolds can be taken with any calipers, these specific directions are for use with either a Harpenden or Lange skinfold calipers. As stated previously, directions for using a plastic model calipers may be found in Appendix A.

Triceps

For the triceps measurement, locate the point over the triceps muscle that is exactly halfway between the elbow (olecranon process) and the shoulder (acromion process of the scapula; see Figure 2.8). When you first begin to practice this procedure, use a tape measure to help locate the halfway point. Once you have located this, use a felt pen to draw a 1- to 2-inch horizontal line to mark the point. Then draw a vertical line through the center of the horizontal line. Now, firmly grasp the skin on either side of the vertical line between the left thumb and forefinger (or the right, if you're left-handed) and lift up the skin with its underlying fat tissue. The horizontal line should be 1/2 inch below your thumb and forefinger. As you grasp the skin, it is important that you not have muscle tissue in your skinfold. To prevent this from occurring, have the athlete make a fist. When the triceps muscle is contracted, you should not be able to feel any muscle tissue in the skinfold.

Once you are sure that you have the correct site and that you don't have any muscle tissue in the skinfold, have the athlete relax the arm;

then take the calipers in your right hand and open the "jaws." Place the contact surfaces 1/2 inch below the fingers of your left (or right) hand. The idea is to position the caliper jaws on the horizontal line at the point of the fold where a true double thickness of fat exists. This will be approximately midway between the crest and base of the skinfold, as shown in Figure 2.9.

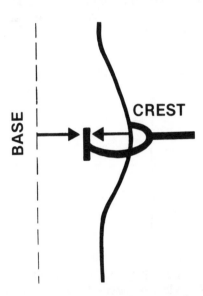

Figure 2.9. Position the calipers at the point of the fold where a true double thickness of skinfold fat exists, which is approximately midway between the crest and the base of the skinfold.

Now slowly release the lever on the calipers so that the jaws are able to exert their full tension on the skinfold. The needle on the caliper dial will drop slightly. When the needle stops moving (within 1 to 2 seconds after you release your grip), read the dial to the nearest 0.5 millimeter (Becque, Katch, & Moffat, 1986). Do not release your grip of the skinfold itself. Record the observed value on a score sheet like the Ideal Weight Recording Form on page 17. Then repeat the procedure two more times at the same site so that you can record three consecutive readings.

Calf

Have your athlete position his or her foot on a platform so that the right knee is at about a 90-degree angle. Using a tape measure, determine the part of the calf that has the largest

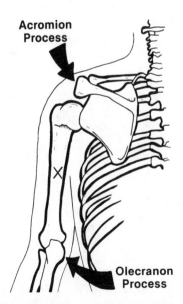

Figure 2.8. Take the triceps skinfold at the midpoint between the acromion process and the olecranon process.

circumference. Use the felt pen to mark this spot with a 1- to 2-inch horizontal line. Now draw a vertical line through the center of the horizontal line (see Figure 2.10). Grasp a skinfold so that your thumb and forefinger are on either side of the vertical line 1/2 inch above the horizontal mark. After making sure that you do not have any underlying muscle, place the jaws of the calipers over the horizontal mark. Once you have located the skinfold site, take the actual measurement in exactly the same way as you did the triceps measurement (see Figure 2.11).

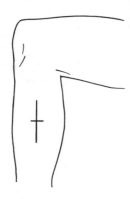

Figure 2.10.   Take the calf skinfold at the level of the largest circumference of the calf. Use horizontal and vertical markings to identify the proper location.

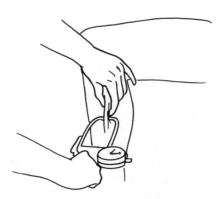

Figure 2.11.   The calf skinfold.

Subscapular

The final skinfold site is the subscapular skinfold (see Figure 2.12). Have the athlete pull his or her shoulders back so that the outline of the scapula (shoulder blade) is exposed. Draw a line with a felt pen along the medial border (the one closest to the spine) of the scapula

to the lower angle of the scapula. Now draw another line at a 45-degree angle to the original line—this line will be along the lower border of the scapula. Cross this line with a short vertical mark. Grasp the skin and fat above the cross mark that you have just made and position the jaws of the calipers over the cross mark. Once you have located the skinfold site, take the actual measurement in exactly the same way as you did the triceps and calf measurements (see Figure 2.13).

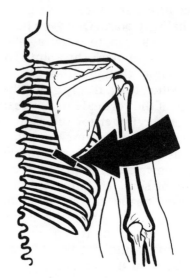

Figure 2.12.   Take the subscapular skinfold over the inferior angle of the right scapula (the bottom right "shoulder blade").

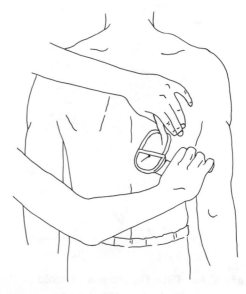

Figure 2.13.   The subscapular skinfold.

Complete the Ideal Weight Recording Form

Once you have finished using the calipers, the most difficult part of measuring body composition is behind you. All that remains to be done is predicting your athlete's ideal weight by following the five steps listed here. The Ideal Weight Recording Form shown below makes this an easy task.

Step 1

Determine the average skinfold values for either the triceps and calf measurements or the triceps and subscapular measurements, and write them in the appropriate spaces on the form. (To determine the average values,

simply add the three measurements for a given skinfold and divide by 3.)

Step 2

Select the appropriate skinfold table (Figure 2.14 or Figure 2.15, pages 18 and 19) on the basis of your athlete's sex and which skinfolds you took.

Step 3

Sum the averages of the triceps and calf or triceps and subscapular skinfolds and place that number on the appropriate line on the Ideal Weight Recording Form. Next, find the sum of the triceps and calf or the triceps and subscapular skinfold averages on the

Ideal Weight Recording Form

Name _____ Age _____ Sex _____

Date _____ Weight _____ lb Height _____ in.

Sport _____ % fat from literature _____ %

Skinfolds

	#1	#2	#3	Average
Triceps	_____ mm	_____ mm	_____ mm	_____ mm
Calf	_____ mm	_____ mm	_____ mm	_____ mm
Subscapular	_____ mm	_____ mm	_____ mm	_____ mm

Sum of the averages of triceps and calf = _____ mm

or

Sum of the averages of triceps and subscapular = _____ mm

Predicted % fat from the appropriate skinfold table = _____ mm

body weight × % fat = fat weight   body weight − fat weight = fat-free weight (FFW)

_____ × _____ = _____   _____ − _____ = _____

$$\text{Ideal body weight} = \frac{FFW}{(100\% - \text{ideal \% fat})}$$

$$= \frac{}{(1.00 -)} = \frac{}{} = \frac{}{}$$

Ideal body weight = _____

Ideal weight prediction _____ lb   Weight to lose/gain _____ lb

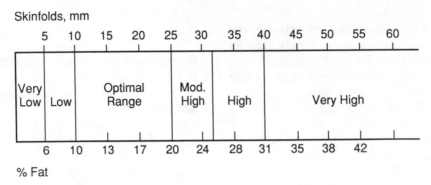

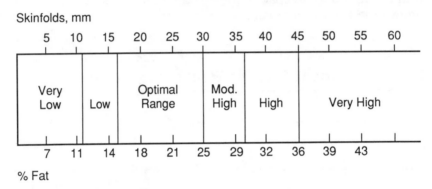

Figure 2.14. Skinfold measurement ranges for the triceps and calf combination. *Note.* From *Measuring Body Fat Using Skinfolds* [Videotape] by T.G. Lohman, 1987, Champaign, IL: Human Kinetics. Copyright 1987 by Human Kinetics. Printed by permission.

corresponding *Skinfold, mm* line of Figure 2.14 (triceps plus calf) or Figure 2.15 (triceps plus subscapular). Draw an imaginary perpendicular line from this sum down to the *% Fat* line. Record this predicted percent fat value in the appropriate place on the recording form.

Step 4

Determine the athlete's fat-free weight (FFW). We will assume that body weight is made up of two compartments, fat weight and lean, or fat-free, weight. The following is an example of how to use the formulas presented in the Ideal Weight Recording Form.

Eric, a middle-distance runner, has 14% body fat and a body weight of 120 pounds.

$$\text{body weight} \times \text{\% fat} = \text{fat weight}$$
$$120 \text{ lb} \times .14 = 16.8 \text{ lb}$$

When we do the rest of the computations, we find that Eric's fat-free weight is 103.2 lb.

$$\text{body weight} - \text{fat weight} = \text{fat-free weight}$$
$$120 \text{ lb} - 16.8 \text{ lb} = 103.2 \text{ lb}$$

Step 5

Now we are ready to determine the athlete's ideal body weight. The formula for doing so follows:

$$\text{ideal body weight} = \frac{\text{fat-free weight}}{100\% - \text{ideal \% fat}}$$

This formula introduces a new term, *ideal percent fat*. Remember, we said that ideal weight is an individual matter, depending upon both the athlete and the sport. Exact values for ideal percent fat are difficult to determine, but research on high school ath-

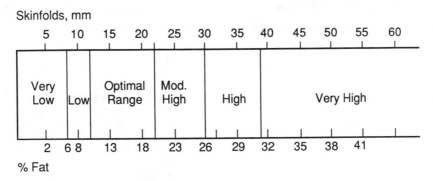

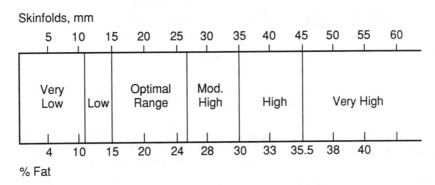

Figure 2.15. Skinfold measurement ranges for the triceps and subscapular combination. *Note.* From *Measuring Body Fat Using Skinfolds* [Videotape] by T.G. Lohman, 1987, Champaign, IL: Human Kinetics. Copyright 1987 by Human Kinetics. Printed by permission.

letes indicates that an athlete's average performance decreases dramatically as body fat increases above 19% in girls and above 10% in boys (McLeod, Hunter, & Etchison, 1983). Other researchers have approached the task of identifying ideal percent fat values by measuring the body composition of successful athletes. We have listed results from some of these studies in Table 2.2. These values can be used as guides for selecting ideal percent fat values to use in the ideal body weight formula. If your sport or activity is not listed, select the sport that comes nearest to your type of activity.

Sample Calculations

Now let's work through an example. Put yourself in the role of Eric's track coach. A completed Ideal Weight Recording Form for Eric is presented in Figure 2.16 on page 21. The blank line calling for "% fat from literature" has "7-12" filled in. This range was selected from Table 2.2 and represents the percent fat range (7% to 12%) for male middle-distance runners. As more research is completed you may have access to more updated ideal percent fat information. When such values are available, by all means use them.

Because of the errors inherent in predicting body composition, it is better to cite a range rather than a single value. We suggest that you use the higher of the two numbers in the range when first computing ideal weight if the athlete is likely to need to lose weight and the lower number if the athlete is likely to need to gain weight. This makes the first goal easier to reach, and it also reduces the likelihood that the athlete will endanger his or her health by losing or gaining too much weight. You can

Table 2.2
Percent Fat Values for Young Athletes
in Various Sports and Activities

Sport (age)	% Fat values Male	Female
Cross-country runners		
(10 yr)	14-15	17-21
Wrestlers		
(11 yr)	13-15	
(17 yr)	11-13	
(16.9 yr)	9-11	
Cyclists		
(13 yr)	10-12	15-20
(15.5 yr)	15-17	16-21
Swimmers		
(15 yr)	10-12	15-17
Tennis		
(15.8 yr)	8-17	16-23
Gymnasts and divers		
(15-17 yr)	8-17	14-20
Track and field		
Middle distance (16-17 yr)	7-12	12-19
Mile walk (16-17 yr)	9-11	15-20
Sprinters and hurdlers		
(16-17 yr)	8-11	13-18
Throwers (16-17 yr)	13-15	22-25
Jumpers (16-17 yr)	8-11	12-18
Ice hockey		
(17-18 yr)	7-10	
Nonathletes		
Prepubescent (9-10 yr)	22-24	26-28
Postpubescent (15-16 yr)	15-17	25-27

Modified from Boileau, Lohman, and Slaughter (1985).

prevent these dangers from occurring by evaluating each athlete's weight change on an individual basis. Procedures for tracking weight modifications are presented later in this chapter and in chapter 11.

As stated previously, the skinfold data in Figure 2.16 demonstrate that Eric is 14% fat. The calculation of his fat weight is also illustrated in the figure. Eric's fat weight is then subtracted from his body weight to calculate his fat-free weight (FFW). Now check to see how the FFW has been entered in the ideal body weight formula.

To complete the ideal body weight calculations for Eric, assume that you believe he will

need to lose some fat weight. Therefore use the higher value in the percent fat range. In this case 12% is entered into the ideal body weight formula presented in Step 5.

$$\text{ideal body weight} = \frac{\text{fat-free weight}}{100\% - \text{ideal } \% \text{ fat}}$$

Subtracting 12% from 100% is the same thing as (1.00 − .12). The results of this subtraction (.88) is shown in Figure 2.16. When the calculations required for the ideal body weight formula are completed, you will have determined that Eric's optimal performance weight should be about 117 pounds. Because Eric's weight is 120 lb, he needs to lose about 3 lb of fat, reducing his body weight to 117 lb for optimal efficiency in cross-country running. Chapter 11 presents some strategies for monitoring the efficacy of the weight loss.

MONITORING FAT LOSS

As indicated in the previous discussions, the skinfold calipers method can be used to predict percent body fat, but many people overlook the fact that skinfold calipers can also be used to monitor subcutaneous fat. If you predict an athlete's body composition and determine that a fat loss goal is necessary, scale weight should not be the only technique used to measure the athlete's progress. You can take skinfold measurements every week or every two weeks to monitor fat losses. Two of the better skinfold sites for tracking subcutaneous fat are the subscapular and calf sites described previously (Roche, Abdel-Malek, & Mukherjee, 1985). If the athlete employs appropriate fat loss procedures, the subcutaneous fat at these two sites should decrease as total body fat is lost, although the exact rate of loss is difficult to predict.

SUMMARY AND RECOMMENDATIONS

You have now learned how to measure and compute body composition and how to calculate ideal weight. But knowing your athlete's approximate ideal weight is only the first step toward getting your athletes to attain their op-

Name _Eric Moore_ Age _16 yrs_ Sex _M_
Date _9/1/88_ Weight _120_ lb Height _62_ in.
Sport _Middle-distance runner_ % fat from literature _7–12_ %

Skinfolds

	#1	#2	#3	Average
Triceps	_8.5_ mm	_9.5_ mm	_9_ mm	_9_ mm
Calf	_7_ mm	_7_ mm	_7_ mm	_7_ mm
Subscapular	____ mm	____ mm	____ mm	____ mm

Sum of the averages of triceps and calf = _16_ mm

or

Sum of the averages of triceps and subscapular = _____ mm
Predicted % fat from the appropriate skinfold table = _14_ %

body wt. × % fat = fat weight   body weight − fat weight = FFW
_120_ × _.14_ = _16.8_   _120_ − _16.8_ = _103.2_

$$\text{Ideal body weight} = \frac{\text{FFW}}{(100\% - \text{ideal \% fat})}$$

$$\text{Ideal body weight} = \frac{103.2\ \text{lb}}{(1.00 - .12)} = \frac{103.2\ \text{lb}}{.88} = 117.27\ \text{lb}$$

Ideal body weight = 117 lb

Ideal weight prediction _117_ lb Weight to (lose)/gain _3_ lb

Figure 2.16. Eric's completed ideal weight recording form.

timal weight. Therefore, you must take the following steps:

1. Help your athletes understand the importance of achieving their ideal weight by emphasizing the importance of lean weight.
2. Utilize body composition assessment procedures rather than just scale weight to emphasize the importance of lean weight to your athletes.
3. Educate your athletes to eat and drink properly to achieve their ideal weight safely and to maintain high energy levels.

In the remaining chapters, we will help you understand how athletes can achieve these goals. One simple way to help athletes achieve their weight control goals is to share this book with them.

Chapter 3
The Balanced Diet

Helping your athletes eat balanced diets requires you to teach them some specific knowledge and skills. Coaches and their athletes must recognize that a balanced diet involves both caloric balance and nutrient balance. Both of these topics are introduced in this chapter. In the nutritional components section of this book, the individual elements of a balanced diet are more fully discussed.

CALORIC BALANCE

A *calorie* is a unit of energy. Technically, a calorie is the amount of energy that it takes to raise the temperature of a gram of water one degree centigrade. The energy that is contained in food is measured in *kilocalories*. The prefix "kilo" means that there are a thousand calories in one kilocalorie. For example, the kilocalories contained in potatoes prepared in different ways are presented in Table 3.1. Several abbreviations for the term kilocalories are common. These include kcal, kcalories, and Calories with the C capitalized. Nutritionists may also use kilojoules (kJ) to mea-

sure the energy contained in food. One calorie equals 4.18 kilojoules. Throughout this book we use the abbreviation *kcal* in tables and figures.

To understand the concept of caloric balance you must recognize that every activity a person performs has an energy requirement that can be expressed in kilocalories, as Table 3.2 shows. Even when you are lying as still as possible, many body functions are taking place to keep you alive.

Some activities require more energy, and thus more kilocalories than others. In addition, all of the foods we eat contain energy. Some foods contain more energy, and thus more kilocalories than others. The fact that the energy value of foods we eat and the energy costs of the body's activities can both be measured in terms of kilocalories forms the basis of the caloric balance concept. The relationship between kilocalories and body weight is frequently introduced by using drawings of a balance scale like the one in Figure 3.1. In this figure, the food on the right-hand side of the scale depicts the kilocalorie content of the foods an individual eats. When that total equals the individual's caloric expenditure,

Table 3.1
Caloric and Nutrient Content for Potatoes Prepared in a Variety of Ways

Type (100 grams)	Kcal	Protein (grams)	Fat (grams)	Carbohydrate (grams)
Baked in skin	93	2.6	0.1	21.1
Boiled in skin	76	2.1	0.1	17.1
French fried	274	4.3	13.2	33.1
Mashed with milk and butter	93	1.9	3.2	14.5
Potato chips	568	5.3	39.8	50.0
Potato salad	99	2.7	2.8	16.3

Table 3.2
Caloric Costs of Daily Activities
for Individuals of Varying Weights

Activity	Kcal per minute		
	110 lb	150 lb	190 lb
Billiards	2.1	2.9	3.6
Carpentry	2.6	3.5	4.5
Circuit training	9.3	12.6	15.9
Cooking (males)	2.4	3.3	4.1
Cooking (females)	2.9	3.1	3.9
Eating (sitting)	1.2	1.6	2.0
Sitting quietly	1.1	1.4	1.8
Running (9 min/mile)	9.7	13.1	16.6
Running (6 min/mile)	13.9	17.3	20.8

the kilocalorie cost of the daily activities depicted by the sporting equipment, the individual is said to be in caloric balance.

NUTRIENT BALANCE

Unfortunately, most people, including athletes, do not look beyond caloric balance as they adjust their diets to lose weight. These people fail to realize that food must do more than just fulfill energy requirements; it must also provide the body with many nutrients. If an athlete does not obtain sufficient quantities of nutrients, such as vitamins and minerals, well-being and performance potential may suffer. Consequently, athletes are faced with two tasks: First, they must eat enough food to obtain the appropriate number of calories to fuel their normal daily activities as well as the extra energy requirements of training and performance. (For some athletes, energy

for growth is also a consideration.) Second, athletes must select foods not only for their caloric content, but for their nutrient content as well. More information about specific nutrient requirements is presented in chapters 6 through 10.

Although it is important to understand the relative contributions of specific nutrients, it is not practical for you to plan your athletes' diets around the nutrient content of specific foods. Adding up every milligram of the various vitamins and minerals that are found in sandwiches, casseroles, fruits, vegetables, and other foods would be quite an impossible task. Instead, use your knowledge about nutrients to help athletes make selections from the four basic food groups.

The Four Basic Food Groups

To simplify the task of selecting foods to achieve a balanced diet, nutritionists have divided foods into four basic groups. By selecting a specified number of foods from each of the four groups, an individual can ensure a balanced diet. These four food groups, as well as the required number of daily servings for each of them, are presented in Table 3.3. The number of servings from the milk and meat groups varies with the athlete's age and the type of training he or she is participating in. This is because these two groups are important sources of protein, and the body requires more protein during periods of physical growth.

Low Nutrient Foods

Frequently, uninformed athletes disregard the concept of nutrient balance and go on low-

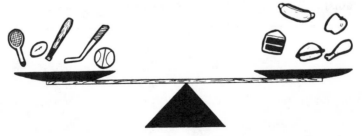

Figure 3.1. If body weight and body composition remain constant, the number of kilocalories in the food eaten will equal the number of kilocalories of energy expended.

Table 3.3
The Four Basic Food Groups

Food group	Servings per day
Milk	
1 c milk, yogurt, or calcium equivalent (1½ oz or 45 g cheddar cheese; 1 c pudding; 1¾ c ice cream; 2 c cottage cheese)	3 for children 4 for adolescents 2 for adults
Meat	
2 oz cooked, lean meat, fish, poultry, or protein equivalent (2 eggs; 2 oz or 60 g chedddar cheese; ½ c cottage cheese; 1 c dried beans or peas; 4 T peanut butter: 2 oz nuts)	2 3-4 for athletes in heavy strength training program
Fruits and vegetables[a]	
½ c cooked or juice 1 c raw	4, including 1 from the vitamin C group, 1 from vitamin A group
Grains	
Whole-grain bread; 1 tortilla; 1 c whole-grain cereal; ½ c cooked cereal, rice, pasta, grits	4

[a]If additional kcal are necessary for additional energy, increase the number of fruit and vegetable servings.

calorie diets where the major concern is that caloric intake not exceed some predetermined value. With this type of diet, an athlete may skip breakfast and eat very little lunch so that he or she can indulge in a high-calorie snack like an ice cream sundae, a piece of pie, or a bag of potato chips. These types of snacks are sometimes called *junk foods* or *empty calories*. This means that the foods contain calories but provide relatively little nutrient value. Another term used to describe such foods is *low-nutrient-density* foods, because so few nutrients are found in each calorie. For example, a candy bar contains so much sugar

and fat that even though peanuts appear in the ingredient list, it is a poor source of protein.

Preparation

The way a food is prepared influences its nutrient density. For example, a raw potato has a relatively high nutrient density (see Table 3.4), because a single potato containing only 100 kilocalories provides 50% of the U.S. Recommended Daily Allowance (RDA) of vitamin C, as well as a number of other nutrients. But depending upon how the potato is prepared, varying amounts of vitamins, minerals, and water are lost. Potato chips, for example, are low in water content and vitamins but high in fat. Therefore they are high in kilocalories, as one gram of fat equals about 9 kilocalories. Due to processing, many water-soluble vitamins are lost. This combination of increased fat content and decreased nutrient content makes potato chips a low-nutrient-density food and a poor choice to fulfill the fruits and vegetables requirement.

Table 3.4
Comparison of Nutrient Density
for Raw Potatoes and Potato Chips
(Percentage of US RDA)

Nutrient	Raw potatoes 100 kcal	Potato chips 100 kcal
Fat	0.1 g	10.0 g
Carbohydrates	21.0 g	15.0 g
Protein	5%	2%
Thiamine	10%	2%
Niacin	11%	4%
Vitamin B$_6$	9%	7%
Vitamin C	50%	10%
Iron	5%	2%

Table 3.1 (p. 23) presented a slightly different picture of the various types of potatoes. An athlete who eats the same quantity (100 grams or about 3 ounces) of the various potato products consumes vastly different amounts of kilocalories, carbohydrates, fats, and proteins. Essentially, cooking the potato in fat, as

is done with french fries and potato chips, increases the caloric content but decreases the relative amount of carbohydrate and eliminates many nutrients.

Nutritional Deficiencies

If the athlete is training hard and losing water-soluble vitamins and some minerals in sweat and urine but is not replacing these lost nutrients because just calories, not nutrients, are being counted, the athlete runs the risk of depriving his or her body of optimal nutrition. Certainly a diet of low-nutrient-density foods increases this risk. To avoid such a risk, athletes should be counseled to balance their nutrient as well as their caloric intake. They can accomplish this by selecting low-fat foods from the four food groups. Typically the goal for most athletes is to consume 65% of their calories as carbohydrate, 15% as protein, and only 20% as fat. Specific information about how to achieve this balance is presented in chapters 11 and 14.

SUMMARY AND RECOMMENDATIONS

You have now learned that a balanced diet involves more than just balancing caloric intake against caloric expenditure. You also know that your athletes must select foods high in nutrients. Now you must take the following steps:

1. Help your athletes recognize that nutrients, as well as kilocalories, are important when selecting foods.
2. Inform your athletes about the four food groups.
3. Educate your athletes as to which foods from the four food groups are high in nutrients.

In addition, it is important for you to help your athletes recognize that kilocalories obtained from foods high in carbohydrates are more advantageous for the athlete in training. The information presented in the next chapter should help you understand the critical relationship between a high-carbohydrate diet, optimal performance, and weight control.

Chapter 4

The Fuel Foods:
Carbohydrates
and Fats

As you learned in chapter 3, a well-balanced diet consists of a variety of foods. Some of these foods have the primary responsibility of providing fuel for the engine-like cells of the body, while others furnish vitamins, minerals, and other essential nutrients. Although fats, carbohydrates, and protein can all serve as fuel foods, only fats and carbohydrates provide energy at a rate capable of sustaining the requirements of physical activity. Because chapter 5 explores how energy is released from foods, this chapter sets the stage by focusing on the chemical composition of fats and carbohydrates, some of the factors that regulate the availability of these fuel foods, and some of the physiological and psychological effects associated with inadequate fuel supplies.

CARBOHYDRATES

The word *carbohydrate* describes the structure of the class of foods commonly known as sugars and starches. All carbohydrates are made up of carbon, hydrogen, and oxygen molecules. Usually, hydrogen and oxygen are present in the same two-to-one proportion as found in water. A German chemist, C. Schmidt, combined the words *carbo* (for carbon) and *hydrate* (for water) to name this class of foods. There are three basic groups of carbohydrates, which differ according to the relative size and complexity of the molecules: simple sugars, disaccharides, and complex carbohydrates.

Simple Sugars

The smallest carbohydrates are the simple sugars, or *monosaccharides*. Glucose, dextrose, and fructose are three monosaccharides often listed on ingredient labels of packaged food. Each of the simple sugars has a slightly different chemical structure; the chemical structure of glucose is diagrammed in Figure 4.1 to help you visualize the relationship between simple sugars and more complex carbohydrates. The *C*s represent carbon molecules, the *H*s hydrogen, and the *O*s oxygen. The lines connecting the carbon, hydrogen, and oxygen atoms represent energy-containing bonds. The double line on the top carbon represents a double bond and more energy. The energy

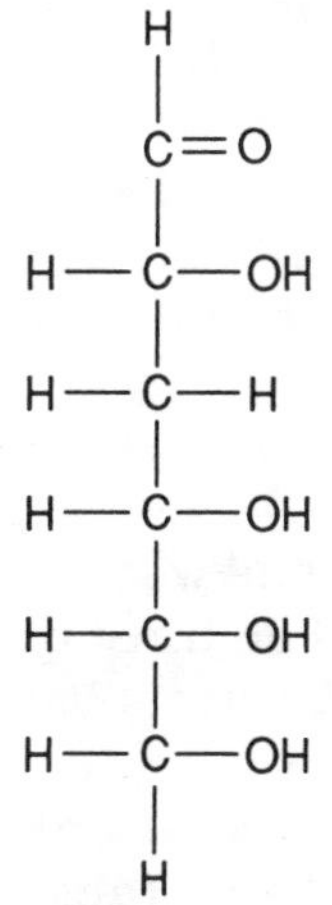

Figure 4.1. The chemical structure of glucose, a monosaccharide.

in these bonds was trapped by plants from light via the process of photosynthesis. Chapter 5 describes how the body unleashes this energy to support life and physical activity.

Disaccharides

The linking up of two monosaccharides results in the formation of a *disaccharide*. Common table sugar, or sucrose, is a disaccharide made from the linking of fructose and glucose. Lactose is the disaccharide found in milk, and it results from the linking of galactose and glucose. Maltose, another disaccharide, is found in products like corn syrup, malted breakfast foods, and malted milk.

Complex Carbohydrates

Strings of several monosaccharides are known as *polysaccharides*. The two types of dietary or plant polysaccharides discussed in this book are starch and fiber. Starch is the carbohydrate found in vegetables such as potatoes, corn, and legumes. The term complex carbohydrate is very descriptive of plant starch because it has been estimated that the number of simple sugar groups in a starch molecule may range from 300 to more than 1,000. Grain and cereal products are also excellent sources of starch.

The second type of polysaccharide is dietary fiber, or roughage. Due to its chemical structure, fiber is not digested and is not a source of calories. For this reason, athletes interested in losing weight need to be sure to incorporate sources of dietary fiber into their diets (see chapter 11).

Though it seems relatively easy to discuss these types of carbohydrates as separate components, in the real world, food products contain mixtures of all three types. For example, many breakfast cereals list all three types of carbohydrates as ingredients. A summary of this information taken from a typical breakfast cereal is included in Table 4.1. Other carbohydrate sources, such as muffins, also contain a wide array of carbohydrates, as illustrated here. Items in italics are carbohydrates.

Table 4.1
Carbohydrate Information for a Breakfast Cereal

Carbohydrate source	Cereal and fruit	With ½ cup vitamin A and D-fortified skim milk
Starch and related carbohydrates	13 g	13 g
Sucrose and other sugars	11 g	17 g
Dietary fiber	5 g	5 g
Total carbohydrate	29 g	35 g

Commercial Muffin Mix

Ingredients: Bleached enriched flour (*wheat flour, malted barley flour*, niacin [A and B vitamins], iron, thiamine mononitrate [vitamin B_1], riboflavin [Vitamin B_2]), *blueberries, sugar*, animal and/or vegetable shortening, *modified corn starch*, salt, *wheat starch*, artificial flavor.

Glucose and Glycogen

To learn how carbohydrates actually become fuel to meet our bodies' energy needs, we must examine what happens to foods that contain carbohydrates once they enter the body. Disaccharides and polysaccharides are too complex to be absorbed from the intestine directly into the bloodstream, so the digestive enzymes first have to break them into monosaccharides, or simple sugars. These monosaccharides can then enter the bloodstream. Of all the simple sugars, only glucose can be directly used by the cells. So when the blood passes through the liver, the liver converts the other simple sugars to glucose.

Because having high levels of glucose in the bloodstream (as occurs in uncontrolled diabetes) is unhealthy, and because cells can "burn" glucose only when it is inside them, glucose must enter the cells. A hormone called *insulin* plays an important role in this process. After carbohydrates are consumed, the elevated glucose levels in the blood signal the pancreas to release insulin. Insulin helps carry glucose into all cells except brain cells; glucose can enter these without the presence of insulin.

As the glucose is taken into cells, some is used for energy (see chapter 5) and some is stored as a polysaccharide called *glycogen*. Just as there is a limit to how much fuel you can put into your car's tank, there is also a limit to the amount of glucose the glycogen tanks can hold. If the glycogen stores are filled, excess glucose is converted to fat and stored in fat (or adipose) cells, as depicted in Figure 4.2.

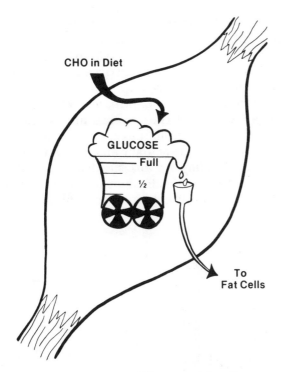

CHO in Diet

GLUCOSE

Full

½

To Fat Cells

Figure 4.2. Excess carbohydrates spill over into the fat storage tanks.

The primary glycogen storage sites are in the muscles and the liver, which have a finite capacity for storing glycogen. Unfortunately, athletes who are unaware of this may overindulge in carbohydrate foods in the belief that they are storing quick energy, when in reality they may be storing fat. Following the dietary guidelines presented in chapter 14 should help to prevent this situation from occurring. In addition, physical training increases the muscles' capacity for glycogen storage—the muscles of a trained athlete are capable of holding nearly twice as much glycogen as those of an untrained individual. But even this increased storage capacity provides enough energy for only 2 to 3 hours of intense exercise. So if you want your athletes to be capable of maximal effort for an entire race or throughout a whole tournament, be sure to encourage them to consume high-carbohydrate foods but not to exceed their caloric needs.

Muscle Glycogen

This glycogen is very important to athletes because almost all of the carbohydrate used during athletic events comes from these glycogen stores. One extremely important aspect of muscle glycogen is that this fuel is stored "on-site" directly in the muscle cells. In other words, muscle glycogen is stored very near to where it will be used.

The glycogen that is stored in a given muscle may be utilized as a fuel only by that specific muscle. Once glucose enters most cells, it cannot leave as glucose, and for this reason, glycogen cannot be shared with other muscles or nerve cells. Liver cells are the major exception to this rule; the liver has the unique ability to convert glycogen back to glucose that can be released into the blood. This makes liver glycogen very important to the exercising athlete, as is explained in the following section.

Liver Glycogen

As mentioned previously, insulin allows the liver as well as the muscles to store glucose as glycogen. Nerve cells, particularly those in the brain, depend on blood glucose for their fuel supply—they do not store glucose and do not readily use fat as fuel. Thus, it is critical that glucose levels be maintained. When the blood glucose level drops (a condition known as hypoglycemia), the nervous system is unable to function optimally. If you have ever skipped breakfast and lunch on the same day, you have experienced some effects of decreased glucose supplies to the brain. When your nerve cells are deprived of their optimal fuel supply, you are less able to concentrate, and you become irritable and lethargic (see Figure 4.3). These symptoms can be even more pronounced in an endurance athlete who does not continually replace liver glycogen by regular carbohydrate consumption. (In fact, the term *bonking* is used by distance cyclists to describe the disorientation and fatigue resulting from hypoglycemia).

The typical sedentary individual and the knowledgeable cyclist do not normally experience hypoglycemia. If the liver has adequate glycogen stores, the liver can convert glycogen back to glucose and release it into the blood if necessary, thereby maintaining blood glucose levels for the brain to use. The liver releases glucose only when blood glucose levels fall below the optimal range. Decreasing blood glucose levels not only signal the release of stress hormones, which cause the liver to break down its glycogen, but also signal the pancreas to stop releasing insulin. At rest, all cells except nerve cells need insulin to use glucose; stopping the release of insulin is the body's way of sparing blood glucose for the nerve cells.

During exercise, even a decrease in insulin release does not prevent muscles from utilizing blood glucose as a fuel. Consequently, intense exercise can deplete both the liver and muscle glycogen storage tanks. This depletion

and the subsequent potential for impaired performance can be minimized by understanding the role of fat as a fuel. To prepare you for the discussion of fat metabolism in chapter 6, let's examine the class of foods known as fats.

FATS

Most of the fats that you eat are transported to specialized cells in the body, known as adipose tissue cells, where they are stored as *triglycerides*. Trigylcerides are composed of three fatty acid molecules joined to a glycerol backbone (see Figure 4.4). Fats contain large amounts of carbon and hydrogen and a relatively small amount of oxygen. They also have a great many bonds and contain a great deal of energy. For example, carbohydrate contains about 4 kilocalories of energy per gram, while fat contains about 9 kilocalories of energy per gram. Consequently fat is said to have a high-calorie density. Because they contain so many calories and because excess body fat can detract from physical performance potential and negatively affect the physical appearance of athletes, dietary fats have a bad reputation. Fats, however, are actually an important source of energy. They are also needed for building cell membranes, skin, hormones, and other structural and functional components of the body.

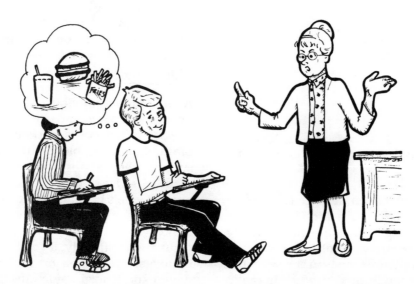

Figure 4.3.   Without adequate carbohydrate intake, maintenance of blood glucose concentration is impossible.

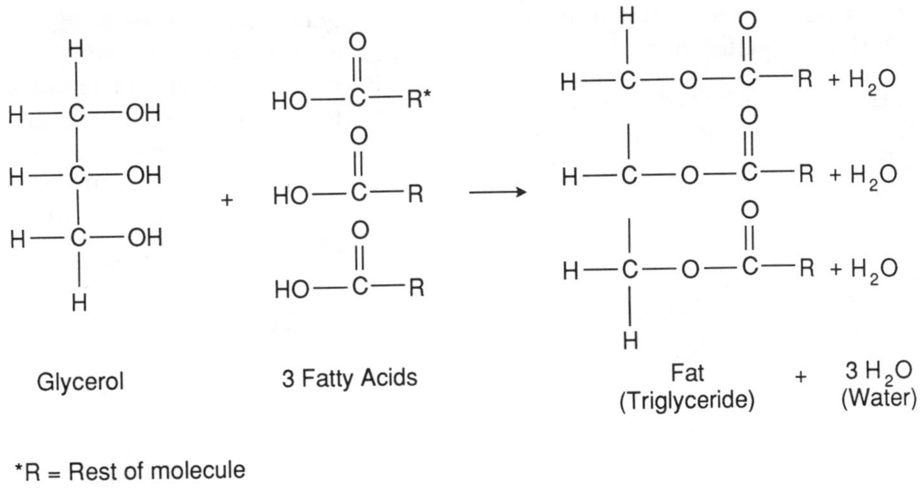

*R = Rest of molecule

Figure 4.4. A triglyceride is made up of three fatty acids and a glycerol backbone.

Slow Sources of Energy

Whereas muscle glycogen is stored in the muscle close to where it will be used, to use fats as fuels your body must mobilize the free fatty acids from the triglycerides in the adipose cells, transport them to the active muscle, transport them across the cell membrane, and finally burn them to release energy. Even if there were no other differences between the energy-releasing processes for fats and for carbohydrates, the difference in storage locations would profoundly affect the rate at which each can be processed to release energy. Although fats do not provide energy as quickly as carbohydrates do, more energy can be stored as fat. Thus, fats provide an important fuel source for prolonged activities. In fact, research with marathon runners shows that performance can be substantially improved if fats can be mobilized and used as fuel early in a race so that the glycogen stores can be saved for later (Costill, Dalsky, & Fink, 1978).

Saturated Versus Unsaturated Fats

Not all fats are equally valuable as energy sources. Fats derived from animal sources as well as those derived from coconut oil and palm oil have a high percentage of saturated fats. The term *saturated* indicates that all possible sites for hydrogen molecules are filled or saturated with hydrogen molecules. Fats derived from most plant sources, however, are unsaturated. Chemically, this means that one (monosaturated) or more (polyunsaturated) of the hydrogen sites are unfilled, and that in each instance there is one or more carbon-to-carbon double bonds. Diets high in saturated or animal fats are thought to lead to increased incidence of atherosclerosis and cardiovascular disease. Therefore, the American Heart Association strongly recommends that we reduce the amount of saturated fat in our diets.

As a coach, you should encourage athletes to minimize their consumption of fats, so that fats do not account for more than 20% to 30% of their diets, but *not* to totally exclude them. Also emphasize that vegetable oils and plant fat sources are best. Take particular care to convey the dangers associated with high-saturated fat diets to athletes involved in weight gain programs (see chapter 13). Eating a diet high in saturated fats not only reduces the athlete's consumption of carbohydrates, it fosters poor lifetime eating habits as well.

SUMMARY AND RECOMMENDATIONS

You have now learned that carbohydrates and fats are the primary fuel foods for physical activity. You also understand that energy stored in the bonds of the carbohydrates and fats must be released to supply the power for muscle contractions. Therefore, it is important that you take the following steps:

1. Emphasize that carbohydrates and fats, not proteins, are the important fuel foods for athletes.
2. Help your athletes begin to identify good food sources for carbohydrates and unsaturated fats.
3. Encourage them to read labels. By doing so, they become aware of the ingredients in various foods and become more able to determine if a food contains carbohydrates and unsaturated fats.

Chapter 5
The Energy Systems

The athletically trained human body is much like a high-performance sports car: It requires high quality fuel. Most of the metabolic machinery within the body has been finely tuned to do one thing: rapidly convert food molecules to a useful form of energy to power the development of muscular tension.

The metabolic requirements of physical activity are enormous compared to those of rest. For example, to maintain normal body function at rest requires approximately 1.5 kilocalories per minute for athlete and non-athlete alike. During strenuous exercise, however, energy requirements can exceed 25 kilocalories per minute for extended periods of time (i.e., several hours) in a highly trained athlete. This represents an increase of more than 1,600% over resting levels!

Where does the extra energy needed to power muscular activity come from? How is your body able to increase the rate at which it breaks down food over 16 times above the resting rate? If you were to ask a biochemist these questions, you would very likely get extremely detailed, extremely incomprehensible answers. You would hear about aerobic and anaerobic oxidation of carbohydrates, fats, and proteins; about the phosphorylation of ADP to ATP in the cytoplasm and the mitochondria; about the electron transport chain; and about lots of other complex-sounding processes. If you are like most people, you would pretend to be intensely interested in this lecture, and when it was over would thank the scientist sincerely, walk away shaking your head, and think to yourself, "Gosh, now that sure was useless information." Not to belittle your natural first response to such a discourse, we sincerely believe that understanding at least the essence of the biochemist's

reply is essential if you, as a coach, are to understand the essential aspects of the optimal sports performance diet.

Fortunately for you, we also believe that these answers need not be so complicated as to sound like a foreign language. In fact, in the next few pages we present a very simplified model that accurately describes the interaction of those systems that release the energy that allows us to perform. Our goal in presenting this information is not to make your busy life more complicated than it already is, but rather to provide you with the necessary background information that will enable you to make educated decisions regarding your athletes' diets.

THE ENERGY CURRENCY OF THE CELL

Deep within every cell in your body is a tiny molecule that is used by almost all living things on this planet as a carrier of energy. The molecule is called *adenosine triphosphate* or *ATP*. Because of its central role in the production and application of metabolic energy, it is commonly referred to as the energy "currency" of the cell. The composition of ATP is actually quite simple. It contains four essential parts or groups (see Figure 5.1): an adenosine group connected to three phosphate groups.

As with carbohydrates and fats (discussed in chapter 4), the connections between the atoms of this molecule are composed of energy-containing chemical bonds that, when broken, release their energy. However, the bonds holding the last two phosphate groups onto the molecule are very special "high-energy"

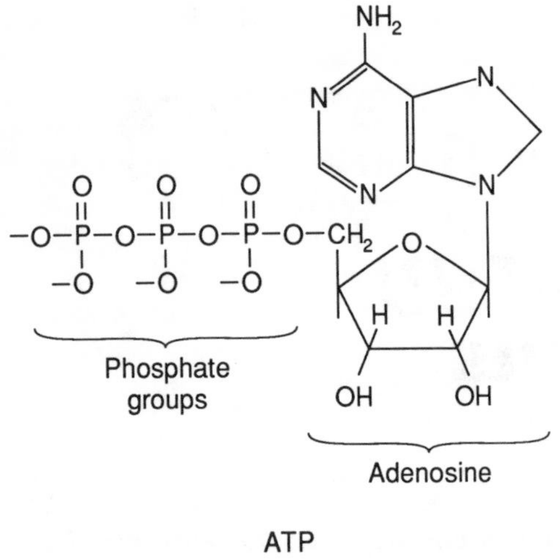

Figure 5.1. ATP, the energy currency of the cell, contains an adenosine group and three phosphate groups.

bonds that liberate more energy when broken than the bond holding the first phosphate group to the molecule. It is the energy in these last two bonds that is used to provide the energy requirements of physical activity (and resting requirements as well).

Hydrolysis

The energy in the molecule is made available when the bond (see Figure 5.2) between the

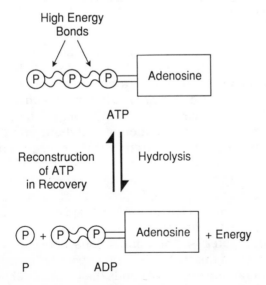

Figure 5.2. Energy is released in hydrolysis when the bond between the last two phosphate groups is broken. ATP is formed when the last phosphate group attaches itself during recovery.

last two phosphate groups is broken, leaving a molecule of adenosine diphosphate (ADP) and free phosphate (P), and the energy that was in the bond is released. Normally this energy would simply be released as heat energy; this is how the kilocalorie unit is used to measure the amount of energy in food. Our cells, however, are very clever and have developed the capacity to capture the energy released by the hydrolysis of ATP and use it to power other reactions that require energy.

The transfer of energy from one reaction to another is known as *coupling*. In other words, the breakdown of ATP and subsequent release of energy is coupled to reactions that need the input of energy in order to proceed (such as the reactions that power muscular contraction).

Production of ATP

For the food we eat to be used by the muscles (or by any other cell in the body) as a source of energy, it must first be "converted" to ATP. The process of conversion or oxidation of food molecules in our cells can be conceptualized as a sort of biological refining process that is in many respects similar to the refining of gasoline from crude oil (though in reality is quite different). If we let gasoline represent ATP, then our cells take food molecules (crude oil) and refine them to produce ATP (high-test gasoline). The food molecules themselves do not provide any direct energy to the cells, but instead provide the raw materials to make ATP, which, like gasoline in a car engine, is used directly in our biological engines to power all of the metabolic processes of the cell.

Just as different grades of crude oil are used in the gasoline refining process, different grades of food molecules can be oxidized to produce ATP. However, as discussed in chapter 4, of all the myriad foods we eat, only two basic categories serve as significant energy foods: carbohydrates and fats. The third category of food, protein, provides cellular building blocks and is not normally used to any great extent in energy production by the muscle cells. (You can read more about protein in chapter 6.)

If we think of ATP as high-test gasoline that is used to power physical activity, then we can envision the mechanisms that produce it from carbohydrates and fats as miniature refining factories that accept molecules of fat or carbohydrate as raw material and output the refined product: ATP. An important factor in understanding the interplay of ATP production in the muscle cell is that the actual refining machinery consists of chemical substances called *enzymes*, which control the rates of many distinct biochemical reactions that systematically "chop up" fats and carbohydrates, liberating the energy contained in the bonds of these food molecules.

THE ENERGY SYSTEMS

There are three different sources or systems responsible for the production of ATP in the muscle cell: ATP-PC, glycolysis, and aerobic. Each of these "factories" is able to provide energy, in the form of ATP, for muscular activity at a different rate, and each has a different total capacity. In general, the total energy capacity of the three systems is inversely proportional to the rate at which they can provide the energy (see Figure 5.3). This difference in both rate and capacity is the basis for understanding the interplay of energy production during exercise. For example, the peak running speed of over 27 miles per hour that an athlete reaches while running a 100-meter sprint reflects the high rate of energy release from the ATP-PC energy system. The fact that a running speed of 27 miles per hour can be sustained for only a few seconds reflects the limited capacity of the ATP-PC system. On the other hand, well-trained marathoners can run at speeds of around 10 to 12 miles per hour for over 2 hours because although the aerobic

system can release energy only at a low rate, it has a large capacity; therefore, slower running can be sustained for hours.

Not only do the three ATP systems produce energy at different rates and have different capacities, they also have different fuel requirements. In other words, what the athlete eats influences the energy-releasing capabilities of the ATP factories. Consequently, if you are going to give your athletes sound nutritional advice, you must understand some basics about the ATP factories.

The ATP-PC Factory

The fastest of the three energy systems is actually not an ATP production factory as much as it is a special storage form of high-energy substances that are immediately convertible to ATP. Most of these high-energy substances are stored as molecules of phosphocreatine (PC). PC is made of a creatine group connected to a phosphate group by a chemical bond. As the level of ATP begins to decline in the cell during muscular contraction, PC is capable of immediately providing a phosphate group and the energy to convert ADP back into ATP (Figure 5.4). Thus, each PC is the equivalent of one ATP.

Explosive Nature

The ATP-PC system is capable of instantaneously providing ATP to be used to power muscular contractions. Therefore, this system is the immediate energy system of the cell,

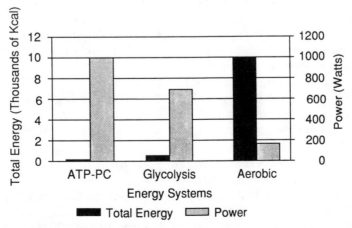

Figure 5.3. The total energy capacity of the three systems is inversely proportional to the rate at which they can provide energy.

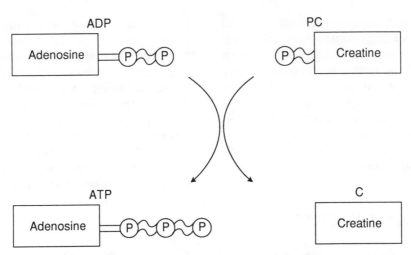

Figure 5.4. As the ATP level declines, PC combines with ADP to resupply ATP.

providing ATP for all activities that are explosive in nature. For example, the energy for a high jump, football line play, and gymnast's vault is provided primarily by the ATP-PC system. Unfortunately, only a relatively small quantity of PC can be stored in the cell, so the ATP-PC system can provide energy for only a few seconds. If an athlete runs several sprints one after another with no rest in between, the sprints will be progressively slower. If rest is allowed, some of the PC can be replaced by the chemical reactions in the aerobic system.

Capacitive Nature

The capacitive nature of the ATP-PC system also makes it very important for providing energy during transition periods when the cell goes from one level of steady-state energy production to a higher level. The basketball player who has been playing a controlled tempo game and suddenly shifts to a fast break offense will immediately need a higher rate of ATP release. Due to its storage capacity, the ATP-PC system can provide this ATP.

The importance of a storage capacity can perhaps best be expressed by a comparison to the production of power in a typical home entertainment stereo system. Each stereo amplifier has a power supply capable of delivering finite amounts of energy at a fixed rate. This would be fine except that the level of the music signal being amplified is not fixed. In fact, music is extremely dynamic—it has many peaks, representing loud passages, separated by valleys, representing quiet passages. To manage the dynamics of musical energy pro-

duction, stereo power amplifiers use large capacitors that store electrical energy. The power supply in the amplifier feeds energy directly to these capacitors, keeping them "topped off." During normal passages, the capacitors are filled by the power supply at a rate equal to the rate at which it is being removed to amplify the music. During brief loud passages, the rate of energy use is much greater than the rate at which the power supply can provide energy. When this happens, the capacitors can immediately release some of their reserve supply to maintain the output of sound. The capacitors are then refilled during the quiet passages by the steady energy production of the power supply.

In the previous analogy, the power supply represents the refinement processes of anaerobic and aerobic metabolism systems that are described on pages 37-39. The capacitors then represent the ATP-PC system. The refinement of food molecules to energy takes time and can proceed only at a finite, fixed rate. However, the energy requirements of the cell during physical activity are incredibly dynamic. These dynamic requirements are sustained by the ATP-PC system, which can provide energy at extremely high rates for short periods of time, and then be "refilled" during periods of lower energy demands.

Limitations

The factors that could potentially limit the production of ATP by the ATP-PC system are the amount of ATP and PC in the cell, and the rate at which PC can be used to convert ADP to ATP. Although the rate of ATP production by the ATP-PC system is very high, the total amount of ATP that it can provide is limited due to the fact that ATP and PC levels in the cell are relatively low. In fact, the ATP-PC system can provide energy for only a few seconds during intense physical activity. However, because extremely intense physical activity requires energy production at an extremely high rate, the ATP-PC system is the major contributing energy system in this instance. This explains why it is possible to sustain extremely high-intensity activity for only a few seconds.

The Glycolysis System

Glycolysis is the process of splitting (refining) a single 6-carbon molecule of glucose into two 3-carbon molecules of pyruvate, which is the link between glycolysis and the aerobic system, and producing two molecules of ATP in the process. Although glycolysis involves several distinct steps, it has been reduced to a single process "box" in Figure 5.5.

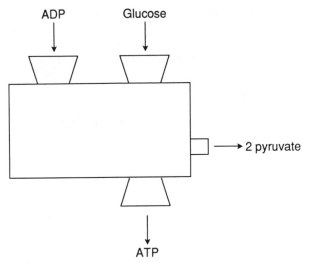

Figure 5.5. Glycolysis is the process by which glucose is refined into pyruvate and ATP.

Aerobic Glycolysis

During the reactions of glycolysis, electrons must be "captured" and removed from the molecules that will ultimately become pyruvate. At rest, or during mild exercise, the rate at which glucose molecules are "chopped up" into pyruvate molecules is relatively slow.

Consequently the electron carriers can easily remove the electrons and take them to the part of the cell where there is ample oxygen from the blood to accept the electrons. When the glycolysis reactions take place at this *slow* rate and enough oxygen is available to accept the electrons, this system is known as *aerobic glycolysis*. The word *aerobic* means with oxygen and refers to the fact that the chain of events required to break down glucose can continue because of the presence of oxygen.

Anaerobic Glycolysis

However, during moderate to extreme exercise, the need for ATP production increases. To meet this need, glucose molecules are chopped up at a *faster* rate. During intense exercise, however, oxygen cannot be delivered fast enough for the electron carriers to keep up with the release of electrons from glycolysis. When this occurs, the reactions that allow glucose to be broken down grind to a halt. Remember that this chopping process is releasing energy to remake ATP. Therefore, if glycolysis stops, so does the athlete. All of these steps would probably occur in less than 10 seconds. In reality, well-trained athletes can perform maximal bouts of exercise for up to one minute and intense exercise for several minutes. How is this possible?

Muscles have an enzyme that allows pyruvate to temporarily accept the released electrons whenever pyruvate is converted to lactic acid. The result is that excess pyruvate is rapidly converted to lactic acid, and glycolysis can continue to produce ATP without relying on the availability of oxygen (as in aerobic glycolysis) to accept the electrons liberated during glycolysis. When oxygen is no longer readily available to accept the electrons released from glycolysis, the term anaerobic glycolysis is used, meaning that the process does not depend on the presence of oxygen.

The combination of the ATP-PC and aerobic systems provides adequate energy for sustained activities. However, these systems fall short of generating the energy necessary for sustained explosive activities. The production of lactic acid through anaerobic glycolysis is absolutely essential for the production of energy by glycolysis during intense exercise. In other words, lactic acid must be produced during high-intensity exercise. If it were not, we would be limited to the capacity of the ATP-PC system and the aerobic system and performance would deteriorate.

Although the production of lactic acid is essential, if it remained in the cell, it would rapidly increase to levels that would inhibit its own formation, halting glycolysis. Fortunately, lactic acid does not remain in the cell but instead rapidly crosses the muscle cell membrane where it is carried away by the blood. This allows glycolysis to continue at high rates, producing lactic acid as it goes, until levels of lactic acid rise to such levels in the blood that it can no longer diffuse out of the cell. When this happens, the rate of glycolytic energy production rapidly decreases. This situation has been experienced by most of us. It is the feeling that comes during the last few yards of a 440-yard dash, a 100-yard freestyle swim, or the final seconds of the finishing sprint in a bicycle race. Lactic acid levels have risen to such a high level that glycolysis cannot produce ATP at a rate sufficient to power continued activity. We are forced to stop even though our spirits may be willing to continue.

Limitations

Limiting factors for glycolysis include the cellular levels of glucose, the special electron carriers, and the activity of the enzymes responsible for converting glucose to pyruvate. In trained athletes, the activity of the glycolytic enzymes is very high. As a result, the glycolytic system is able to rapidly convert glucose to pyruvate, producing ATP in the process. Because glucose molecules are stored directly in the cell in the form of glycogen, and because glycogen can be rapidly broken down to liberate those glucose molecules, the glycolytic energy production system is able to provide ATP at high rates for relatively long periods of time. As indicated previously, the production of lactic acid allows glycolysis to continue temporarily. Glycolytic ATP production can continue until glycogen levels are depleted in the cell or lactic acid accumulates in the cell.

During very intense exercise, lactic acid accumulation usually forces a halt to exercise within 60 to 90 seconds, long before glycogen is depleted from the muscle cells. However, should glycogen levels become low due to prolonged activity; repeated bouts of short, intense activity; or a low-carbohydrate diet, glycolytic ATP production can be affected.

The Aerobic Energy System

The final energy production system is actually two closely linked systems that reside in a cell structure known as the *mitochondria*. Because the extraction of energy from food molecules in the mitochondria requires oxygen, the term "aerobic" energy production is used. A mitochondrion and its aerobic energy processes is diagrammed in Figure 5.6. Notice that both pyruvate (the output of glycolysis) and free fatty acids (FFA) are shown as input.

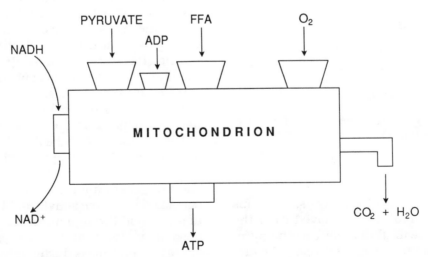

Figure 5.6. The aerobic energy system is made up of two closely linked systems that operate within the mitochondria.

The aerobic energy production system of the mitochondria is capable of breaking bonds in fats and the by-products of glycolysis. However, oxygen is required for these processes to occur.

The usable output of aerobic energy production is ATP, and the by-products (exhaust) of this system are carbon dioxide and water. It is very important to remember that the rate of energy production sustainable by this system is fixed by the availability of oxygen in the cells. The result of this reliance on cellular oxygen levels is that the aerobic system is the *slowest* energy producer of the three systems described so far (see Figure 5.3). However, this system breaks more bonds and thus releases far more of the potential energy in the molecules that it processes. The result is that the amount of energy that the aerobic system can produce is much greater than with glycolysis. If one molecule of glucose goes through glycolysis, two molecules of ATP are produced. If the two pyruvates from that molecule of glucose continue on through the aerobic energy system, 36 molecules of ATP will be produced. Consequently, the aerobic system can provide energy at a relatively slow rate (e.g., enough energy to run at 8 to 12 miles per hour), for extended periods of time (e.g., 2 to 3 hours).

Limitations

Factors that can limit the rate of aerobic energy production include the availability of carbon molecule substrate (derived from glucose and free fatty acids) and the availability of oxygen. Notice that two of the three potential limiting factors (free fatty acids and oxygen) are derived from extracellular sources and must be delivered to the cell during the actual energy production process. It is true that free fatty acids are not essential, as muscle glycogen can provide glucose, but oxygen is essential for the aerobic oxidation of both free fatty acids and carbohydrates. If levels of oxygen in the cell are not sufficient to meet metabolic demands, then the aerobic energy system will not be able to supply the ATP required.

THE BIG PICTURE

On paper it is relatively easy to separate the functioning of the three energy systems, but in real life they do not operate in isolation. Instead, as the level of energy utilization in the muscle cells increases along with the athlete's level of physical exertion, all of the energy production systems increase their output of ATP in an attempt to meet the demands of the active cells.

Steady-State Exercise

Steady-state exercise is, by definition, exercise at a level that can be maintained for prolonged periods of time. The aerobic energy production system is primarily responsible for providing ATP at this level of activity. This is, in fact, very desirable, because the energy production capacity of this system is much greater than that of the ATP-PC or anaerobic glycolysis systems. However, athletic performances often involve energy expenditure at rates that are sustainable for only very short periods. In these situations, the interaction of the various energy systems becomes quite important.

Steady-State Limits

We are now in a position to better understand the relationship between carbohydrate utilization and exercise intensity. During exercise each energy system increases its rate of ATP production until one of two conditions is met:

- The rate of ATP production equals the rate of ATP utilization.
- The energy system becomes limited due to the unavailability of some essential substrate.

Remember, as described above, the ATP-PC system is similar to a storage tank of high-energy phosphates (ATP and PC), while the glycolytic and aerobic systems are processes that actually produce ATP from breaking the bonds of food molecules.

Anaerobic Versus Aerobic Production

The major practical difference between aerobic and anaerobic energy production is that aerobic energy production must rely on extracellular factors. In other words, the factors affecting the rate of energy production by the ATP and glycolytic systems depend only on materials that are stored in the cell. On the other hand, the maximum rate for the aerobic production of ATP is tied to oxygen availability, an essential element that is provided by extracellular delivery systems.

Surges and Spurts

During sports and other physical activities, the energy demands of individual muscle cells are in a state of flux. Consider the example of a marathon runner, who may seem like the epitome of steady-state exercise. But this runner must climb hills, change speeds to meet challenges from other runners, and sprint at the end of the race. All of these surges and spurts require rapid adjustments in the rate of ATP production by the active muscle tissue. These adjustments in cellular energy production must occur in a much shorter time frame than can be accommodated by the cardiovascular oxygen delivery system. This means that the anaerobic energy systems (ATP-PC and anaerobic glycolysis) are extremely important, whether your athletes are soccer players making breakaway tackles or baseball players running down a fly ball.

Carbohydrates Are the Fuel

It is now easy to see that the amount of energy produced by the ATP-PC system and anaerobic glycolysis becomes more and more important as exercise intensity increases and

oxygen becomes even more limiting to the aerobic system. The result is that anaerobic ATP production is essential for all physical activity—especially for the high-intensity, intermittent activity associated with technique sports like basketball and high-intensity endurance sports like running and cycling. Because carbohydrate-derived glucose is the only food substance that can be oxidized (refined) to produce ATP anaerobically, it is the essential fuel for an athletic performance.

SUMMARY AND RECOMMENDATIONS

Understanding the systems that make energy available to the athlete is critical to appreciating the importance of carbohydrate as a fuel for optimal physical performance. Now that you have read this chapter you should understand the interplay between the three energy-releasing systems and their associated performance potentials. But just reading and understanding this material is not enough. Now you must take the following steps:

1. Help your athletes realize that carbohydrates are key fuel foods.
2. Begin to familiarize your athletes with foods that are good sources of carbohydrate as well as nutrients.

The next section of this book contains information that you can use to help your athletes make good food choices. In the final section of the book we present the specifics of a high-performance diet.

PART II
Nutritional Components

Chapter 6
Proteins and Amino Acids

For years advertisements in many sport and fitness magazines have claimed that athletes benefit from the use of protein supplements. Because proteins from the meat, milk, cheese, and grain products we eat are used as building blocks for muscles, bones, and other structures in the body, most of these ads have been targeted to body builders and other athletes interested in developing size and muscle mass. Because proteins are actually made up of chains of smaller chemical structures called *amino acids*, an extension of this advertising ploy now finds amino acid supplements, or "aminos," being marketed to football players, weight lifters, and other athletes interested in "bulking up." Some ads suggest that amino acids facilitate endurance performance, and others tout their use to reduce body fat. Do proteins and amino acids really do all of these things? How do amino acids differ from protein supplements? Are there any dangers associated with using protein supplements or "aminos"? In this chapter, we explain what proteins and amino acids are and what they do. We also discuss how much of these substances strength and endurance athletes really need.

THE CHEMICAL COMPOSITION OF PROTEINS

Proteins are very large complex substances that form the structural framework of the body. The substances that control all the chemical reactions in the body (enzymes) are also made of proteins. Thus, physical growth, the repair of damaged tissue, and the regulation of daily body functions could not take place if proteins were not consumed in the diet.

In actuality, proteins are made of strings or chains of smaller substances called amino acids. Each amino acid is made up of carbon, oxygen, hydrogen, nitrogen, and sometimes sulfur atoms. It is the presence of the nitrogen that makes amino acids, and thus proteins, different from carbohydrates and fats.

Essential Amino Acids

Carbon, oxygen, hydrogen, and nitrogen molecules can be sequenced in a number of different ways. Consequently, there are 20 different amino acids (see Table 6.1). Typically,

Table 6.1
The Amino Acids

Essential amino acids	Nonessential amino acids
Histidine[1]	Alanine
Isoleucine	Arginine
Leucine	Asparagine
Lysine	Aspartic acid
Methionine	Cysteine
Phenylalanine	Glutamic acid
Threonine	Glutamine
Tryptophan	Glycine
Valine	Proline
	Serine
	Tyrosine

[1]Essential for children only; nonessential for adults.

43

8 of these are called essential amino acids, essential because the body must have them and cannot make them from other foodstuffs. The remaining 12 are called nonessential because the liver can use carbohydrates, fats, and the nitrogen from essential amino acids to make them. The one exception to this statement is the amino acid called histidine. For children, it is the 9th essential amino acid because the liver cannot make it fast enough to accommodate children's growth needs.

Amino Acid Sources

Amino acids may be found in the proteins of both animals and plants, but the relative amounts and proportions of essential amino acids are not the same in all food sources of protein. Generally speaking, animal sources of protein have all the essential amino acids and have them in a distribution pattern closer to that required by humans than do plant sources. Consequently, we consider animal protein sources as having higher value or quality than plant protein sources. There is *no* difference in the amino acids themselves between plant and animal proteins—only the distribution of the essential amino acids is different.

The Building Blocks of Life

People should eat both plant and animal protein sources so that the correct complement of amino acids is available to manufacture the structural framework for the various cells of our bodies. Amino acids are used to repair these structures and are the major components of enzymes (the chemicals that regulate life processes) and hormones. Without a diet adequate in calories and in the essential amino acids, antibody production, the maintenance of water and acid-base balances, and the manufacture of hemoglobin to transport oxygen would be impaired. Amino acids are vital substances in our diet and have earned the reputation as the building blocks of life. There is, however, considerable debate as to whether athletes need more amino acids or more of certain types of them and whether it is safe for athletes to consume large quantities of amino acids. Before we examine these concerns, let's look at why protein and amino acid supplementation is so attractive to athletes.

THEORY BEHIND SUPPLEMENTATION

There are at least five reasons why athletes try to eat more protein and amino acids than do sedentary individuals. Some of these reasons apply more to strength athletes and others to endurance athletes. Some athletes use amino acids, proteins, or both, as

- a source of building material for large muscles and the component parts of muscles,
- a source of building material for repairing damaged tissues,
- a source of energy for physical activity,
- a technique for stimulating growth factors in the body, or
- a technique for stimulating fat metabolism to help with fat reduction.

Strength Athletes

Because a primary constituent of muscle is protein and 60% to 70% of the protein in the body is in muscle tissue (Lemon, 1987), athletes who want to increase their muscle size and maintain a larger-than-normal muscle mass reason that they need to consume a larger-than-normal amount of protein. Consequently, these individuals are often attracted by the lure of high-protein foods and protein or amino acid supplements as a means of increasing their consumption. Yoshimura (1970), a sport scientist, has suggested that during the first few weeks of training there is an increased need for amino acids to support the synthesis of new structural and functional proteins in the muscles. Increased consumption of amino acids, especially during the initial weeks of training, will meet this hypothesized need. Many athletes take protein supplements for this reason.

Increased Body Weight

Research that has examined the efficacy of increased consumption of protein, amino acids, or both on the weight and size of the strength and power athlete is not very extensive, and the results have been variable. Some researchers (Blanchard, 1972; Sims, 1970) have reported increases in the body weights of high school and college athletes who used protein supplements. However, because body composition was not measured, it is possible that the weight gained was fat weight, not lean weight. Other researchers (Rasch & Pierson, 1962) have noted that their athletes, with or without protein supplementation, gained body weight while on a weight training program.

Laritcheva, Yalovaya, Shubin, and Smirnov (1978), however, observed that when the weight lifters in their study did not consume extra protein, they were in a negative nitrogen balance. (Remember, nitrogen is found in protein.) If the body is losing nitrogen (causing a negative balance), protein is probably not being used to build muscle tissue.

Decreased Body Fat

Some also claim protein supplementation can help reduce body fat through the release of a growth hormone. There is little research relative to the recent claims (Colgan, 1987) that specific amino acids—L-arginine, L-ornithine, and L-lysine—can be used to stimulate the body to release its own growth hormone. (The L prefix before the amino acid refers to an aspect of its chemical structure and indicates that the amino acid can be used by the body. For example, arginine in a different form, R-arginine, cannot be used by the body.) You might have noticed that L-ornithine is not included in Table 6.1. This is because it is not found in protein foods. Rather, it can be manufactured. You will find it in amino acid supplements being marketed to athletes.

The ingestion of these specific amino acids has been shown to stimulate the release of growth hormone (Besset, Bonardet, Roundouin, Descomps, & Passouant, 1982), but there has been no research to ascertain the effects of amino acid-stimulated increases in growth hormone on gains in muscle strength or size. Growth hormone therapy has been used with children who have growth problems, and under these circumstances the injection of growth hormone has, in fact, resulted in increased muscle growth and decreased subcutaneous fat (Tanner, Hughes, Whitehouse, & Carter, 1977). However, athletes are not typically suffering from growth hormone de-

ficiency. The claim that L-arginine and other amino acids can improve muscle mass development and decrease body fat needs considerably more research.

Endurance Athletes

For endurance athletes like marathoners, distance swimmers, and triathletes, large muscle masses would hinder rather than help performance. Therefore, the ads that promote amino acid use for these types of athletes highlight some different features, such as the use of amino acids as a fuel source.

Protein as an Energy Source

In 1842, Von Liebig (cf. Haymes, 1983) first proposed that protein was an important source of energy during physical work, but this claim was challenged by sport scientists who were unable to note increased nitrogen excreted in the urine of exercisers (Durnin, 1978). Remember, nitrogen is a unique component of amino acids. Before the amino acid can be converted to a fat or carbohydrate and serve as a fuel in the aerobic energy system, the nitrogen must be removed. Typically, most nitrogen is removed as urea in the urine. Because nitrogen does not appear to be removed in the urine of exercisers, which suggests that amino acids have not been used by the aerobic energy system, and because only carbohydrates can serve as fuel for anaerobic glycolysis (see chapter 5), carbohydrates have been promoted as the major source of energy for the intense bouts of activity of athletes.

More recently, researchers have demonstrated that proteins are broken down during endurance exercise (Dohm, Tapscott, & Kasperek, 1987; Lemon, 1987). This finding was made possible by modern techniques that can track the loss of urea in sweat (Lemon, 1987), as well as by recognition of other non-urea nitrogen sources in sweat (Alexiou, Anagnostopoulos, & Papadatos, 1979). In other words, scientists learned that nitrogen left over from the conversion of protein to carbohydrate was escaping from the body in the sweat and not just through the urine. In addition, modern research techniques have also allowed scientists to identify increases in non-urea nitrogen sources in the fecal material and urine that occur with exercise (Steenkamp, Fuller, Graves, Noakes, & Jacobs, 1986).

Generally speaking, the research suggests that amino acids serve directly as fuel and indirectly as support mechanisms for the energy-producing chemical reactions of exercise (Brooks, 1987). Also, the more intense the exercise and the longer its duration, the greater the contribution of amino acids to the energy-producing processes. If the exercise requires an intense effort for more than an hour, the energy from the conversion of amino acids to carbohydrates may contribute 10% to 12% of the total energy requirement. So you can see that carbohydrates, not amino acids, should still account for the bulk of an athlete's diet.

Amino Acids for Growth and Recovery

If the athlete has not been consuming enough carbohydrates, the body must use even more amino acids for fuel and for other purposes (Lemon, 1987). This could deprive the body of the amino acids or building blocks necessary for developing new enzymes or muscles in response to training. Because recovery from training also requires amino acids to restore the tissues, athletes must balance their consumption of carbohydrates with the consumption of some amino acids. Once again we see why a balanced diet is so important. Some specifics as to how much protein is necessary to consume the required amino acids are presented later in this chapter.

Fat Mobilization

It has also been proposed that the ingestion of selected amino acids can stimulate the use of fat as a fuel in the muscles, thus sparing the glycogen stores. This has been suggested because growth hormone stimulates fat burning, and L-arginine, L-ornithine, and L-lysine are hypothesized to increase growth-hormone release (Tanner & Whitehouse, 1967). This interesting hypothesis needs further research.

SUGGESTED PROTEIN INTAKE

The National Research Council's recommended values for protein intake (1980) are dependent upon age and the growth that takes place during childhood (see Table 6.2). Please note that

Table 6.2
Protein Values for Various Age Groups

Age	Recommended Daily Allowance (RDA) values (Grams of protein per kg body weight)	Suggested athlete consumption RDA + 50% to 100% (Grams of protein per kg body weight)
1-3	2.2	—
4-6	2.0	3.0-4.0
7-10	1.8	2.7-3.6
11-14	1.0	1.5-2.0
15-18	0.9	1.35-1.8
19-22	0.8	1.2-1.6
Over 23	0.8	1.2-1.6

Derived from National Research Council (1980).

these suggested values assume the consumption of an adequate number of calories. If an individual restricts calories, protein can and will be converted to fuel sources.

Although there is still considerable disagreement among experts as to exactly how much extra protein athletes need, we believe, based on the research presented in the preceding paragraphs, that athletes do have a slightly increased need for amino acids. Our recommendations relative to these needs are presented in the remaining sections of this chapter.

Amount of Protein Needed

The precise desired increase in amino acid consumption for the athlete is uncertain at this time (Williams, 1985). Furthermore, almost no research has been done to examine the protein requirements of athletes during their growth years. Consequently, we suggest that athletes consume 1.5 to 2.0 grams per kilogram (g/kg) of body weight, which is approximately 50% to 100% more than the Recommended Daily Allowance (RDA) for protein. The more intensely the athlete is training, especially if increased muscle mass is a goal, the more likely it is that the 2.0 g/kg level will be necessary. Coaches should remember that most sedentary Americans already consume more than 2.0 grams of protein for each kilogram of body weight each day. Do not interpret the suggestion that athletes need more protein than the RDA requirements call for to mean that young athletes should buy and use expensive amino acid supplements.

We believe that food is a much better way to obtain protein requirements, particularly for the young athlete. For example, an 88-pound (40 kilogram [kg]), 14-year-old athlete's adjusted protein requirement is 60 to 80 grams of protein per day (40 kg × 1.5 to 2.0 g/kg). By eating a tuna sandwich (which contains 20 grams of protein), two pieces of chicken (24 grams), a yogurt snack (8 grams) and drinking 3 glasses of milk (30 grams) throughout the day, the athlete consumes more than 80 grams of protein. Obviously, extraordinary amounts of food are not necessary to fulfill the protein requirement.

Types of Amino Acids Needed

Although the labels on most protein foods, including meats, dairy products, nuts, and grain products, rarely list specific amino acids, many commercial amino acid supplements present the names of specific amino acids as part of their promotional information. Therefore, coaches need to understand how some specific amino acids are used by the body.

Although humans need to consume all of the essential amino acids, much of the research with athletes has demonstrated that three of the amino acids, leucine, isoleucine, and valine, are particularly important in the energy-producing reactions that occur during exercise (Brooks, 1987). These essential amino acids are very important—they make up 35% of the protein in your muscles. As a result, the manufacturers of amino acid supplements often feature these amino acids in their products. Due to the arrangement of the molecules in leucine, isoleucine, and valine, these three are called branched chain amino acids. When your athletes ask you whether they should buy a supplement that features branched chain amino acids, explain that these amino acids are very important, but they can be obtained from food without costly supplementation. For example, one egg, two slices of bread, 1 cup of skim milk, a 3-ounce lean hamburger patty, 2/3 cup of green peas, 1 tablespoon of peanuts, and one 4-ounce serving of low-fat (1%) cottage cheese provides nearly 58 grams of protein and 4.9 grams of leucine. This amount of leucine represents 500% of the RDA requirement for that amino acid.

To ensure that your athletes receive all the essential amino acids in the correct proportion, encourage them to eat high-quality proteins periodically throughout the day. Examples and additional discussion are presented in chapter 14.

Eating Protein Foods

For the body to synthesize new proteins for building new tissues or for recovering from the stress of training, a full complement of the essential amino acids must be available. Though the body has the ability to store extra fats and carbohydrates, there is no storage form for amino acids. If excessive amounts of protein or amino acids are consumed, the nitrogen is removed and the remaining structure is converted to fat or carbohydrate. The excess essential amino acids cannot be stored.

During exercise there is a decrease in the synthesis of new protein as well as an increase in the breakdown of existing protein. After exercise, the situation changes, and there is an increase in the synthesis of new protein. For this synthesis to proceed properly, the correct proportion of the necessary essential amino acids must be available. Because amino acids cannot be stored, athletes can ensure the availability of essential amino acids by ingesting small quantities of high quality proteins in snacks and meals throughout the day. These snacks and meals should be accompanied by ample glasses of water—the kidney needs adequate water to remove the urea from the protein metabolism.

Protein food snacks may also stimulate growth hormone production. For example, an athlete who is trying to gain weight might eat a turkey sandwich (but hold the mayo) as an evening snack. Theoretically, the amino acids in the turkey might stimulate growth hormone release. Growth hormone release occurs naturally during sleep, and the turkey sandwich *may* add to this. At any rate, the turkey sandwich is much less expensive than a collection of amino acid supplements. In addition, whole-wheat bread, a tomato slice, and some lettuce adds some more vitamins and minerals to the athlete's diet.

COMPLEMENTS FOR PROTEIN

The essential amino acids in high-quality protein foods like turkey can best be utilized if adequate carbohydrate calories accompany them. Consequently, many of the available protein or amino acid supplements include substantial quantities of complex carbohydrates. In this combination, the amino acids are spared from being used as fuel so that they may be used to build and repair tissues. This is another good reason to eat food rather than take supplements. The turkey sandwich that we suggested as a protein snack also contains a lot of carbohydrates in the bread and the tomato.

In addition to a high-carbohydrate, low-fat diet, adequate rest and sleep are necessary for optimal amino acid utilization. Athletes who do not get enough sleep or who do not have a fixed routine of sleep, exercise, and eating are not maximizing the body's ability to use amino acids. Spending money on expensive supplements will not correct this problem.

DANGERS OF EXCESS PROTEIN

Unfortunately, many athletes are unaware of the dangers of eating too much protein. Therefore, you need to be familiar with the potential dangers so that you can warn your athletes about them and be alert for any problems.

Cardiovascular Risks

One of the problems with excessive protein consumption is that animal protein sources like red meat, whole milk, eggs, and most cheeses also contain large quantities of saturated fat. High levels of saturated fat have been shown to be related to increased levels of blood fats and cholesterol as well as increased body fat, high blood pressure, and coronary heart disease. Eating large quantities of fat is particularly dangerous if the athlete's family already tends to have high blood pressure or has a history of coronary heart disease. High blood pressure may be further aggravated by the large amount of salt often eaten with animal proteins. Athletes who eat large quantities of animal proteins are not only likely to gain fat

weight, they are also forming poor lifetime eating habits.

Obesity

Because many animal protein sources are associated with high levels of fat, they contain many calories. Unless the diet is low in total energy foods, much of the extra protein, which cannot be stored, will be converted to fat by the liver and stored as fat. Because extra fat is excess baggage and does not contribute to strength, power, or quickness, eating excessive amounts of protein or amino acid supplements only hinders athletic performance.

The typical "fat American" is not the result of an accident nor the product of some foreign virus; rather, obesity is a reflection of poor eating habits and lack of physical activity. Because sport places a premium on physical efficiency and energy management, as a coach you are in an ideal position to foster positive weight control and motivation habits by encouraging your athletes to eat low-fat, high-quality proteins.

Gout

Don't forget "Moose" McGraw (see chapter 1), who experienced his bout with gout from eating too much protein. Brewer's yeast, a component in some protein supplements, and alcohol can also cause gout (the buildup of excessive uric acid in the blood). Not everyone responds to these substances in this fashion, but some do, especially those with a family history of the condition. In a susceptible individual, alcohol, yeast, and the purine content of protein foods may cause the blood uric acid level to rise. If this uric acid crystallizes in the joints, an attack of gout may result.

Dehydration

Another hidden problem associated with protein metabolism is dehydration, or loss of body water. This occurs because the kidneys must use water to form urine to wash out the nitrogen (urea) and other metabolic waste products from protein metabolism. This explains in part why crash diets can result in rapid weight loss.

During the crash dieting, the body's proteins are used for fuel, thereby producing urea. So water is lost as the kidneys remove urea from the blood.

Ammonia-Smelling Sweat

This is probably not so much a problem of eating too much protein as it is of consuming too little carbohydrate and water. If calories are cut or meals skipped because the athletes is busy, the body is less likely to have adequate muscle glycogen. Therefore, muscle and other proteins as well as fats are broken down so that the working muscles can have the fuels they need. The increased nitrogen that has been removed in the process of breaking down amino acids forms ammonia. The increased loss of these nitrogen wastes in the sweat may cause the ammonia-like smell.

Calcium Deficiency

There is some evidence (Allen, 1982) that increased dietary protein leads to elevated calcium excretion. This study was completed with sedentary subjects, but low bone mass is already a problem for some female athletes. More research is needed to determine if suggestions for increased calcium intake along with protein intake are necessary.

SUMMARY AND RECOMMENDATIONS

Although athletes probably do need more protein than do their sedentary counterparts, a diet with 12% to 15% of the calories coming from high-quality protein sources can easily supply the necessary essential amino acids. The consumption of large quantities of protein and amino acid supplements is not necessary. To help your athletes derive the greatest benefits from protein consumption, you should take the following steps:

1. Encourage your athletes to consume small quantities of high-quality, low-fat protein four to six times throughout the course of the day (including 30 to 60 minutes before and after workouts).
2. Suggest that your athletes eat food rather than take supplements because the supplements are expensive. In their concentrated form, the supplements may also promote excessive consumption.
3. Inform your athletes that by eating food forms of protein they will also be getting carbohydrates, which facilitate the body's use of protein.
4. Insist that your athletes drink plenty of water. This helps the kidneys clear nitrogen and helps prevent dehydration.
5. Plan training programs that allow time for recovery.
6. Educate your athletes about the importance of rest and sleep. They should know that protein supplements cannot make up for poor sleep habits.

Your efforts to educate your athletes relative to these concepts serve as the base for their "nutritional conditioning"—a part of their training that is just as important as their physical conditioning. This education will not only help your athletes play better, it's likely to help them develop eating habits that enable them to live longer and happier lives.

Chapter 7
Vitamins

The word *vitamin* means vital. Vitamins are organic substances that are essential in minute quantities for specific chemical reactions in cells to occur. Because cells cannot manufacture these substances, they must be included in the food we eat.

Some of the vitamins are *fat soluble* (A, D, E, and K) and therefore are absorbed along with fat from the stomach and intestines. Fat-soluble vitamins are readily stored in the body and excessive supplementation of them can lead to vitamin toxicity. In other words, the body can actually be poisoned by too much. For example, an athlete who overdoses on vitamin A could experience thickening of the skin, headaches, and increased susceptibility to disease, and excessive amounts of vitamin D may result in vomiting, diarrhea, muscular weakness, and kidney damage.

It is more difficult to take too much of the *water-soluble vitamins* (the B complex and vitamin C), because excesses of these vitamins are lost in sweat, urine, and other fluids. Recently, however, some detrimental side effects of taking extreme quantities (megadoses) of the water-soluble vitamins have been reported (Rudman & Williams, 1983). These side effects for vitamin C overdose include nausea, diarrhea, kidney stones, and hypoglycemia, while numbness and paralysis are associated with megadoses of the B vitamins.

The measurement units typically used to quantify vitamin doses vary somewhat. For some vitamins the *International Unit* (IU) is utilized. For others, milligrams (mg) are used to quantify the doses. Table 7.1 summarizes the U.S. Recommended Daily Allowances for some fat-soluble and water-soluble vitamins. It also outlines some of the *good* food sources for meeting the daily requirements for each of the vitamins. The word good is emphasized to highlight the fact that two criteria were met before foods were listed as being a good source for a given vitamin:

- The food had to have a high concentration of the vitamin.
- The food had to have a low fat content.

We believe that the second criterion is necessary because many foods that are high in some of the fat-soluble vitamins are also high in fat. For example, a cup of whole milk provides 350 IU of vitamin A, but nearly 50% of its calories are fat calories. Skim milk, on the other hand, has less than 3% of its calories as fat calories but contains only a trace (10 IU) of vitamin A. Consequently milk is not listed as a good food source for vitamin A. Because carbohydrates are the body's preferred fuel, Table 7.1 presents those high-carbohydrate, low-fat foods that are also high in the specific vitamin.

FUNCTIONS OF VITAMINS

Vitamins are involved in the formation of red blood cells, the building of bones, and protein metabolism. Some vitamins act as co-enzymes for the energy-releasing chemical reactions of the body, but the vitamins themselves are not a direct source of energy. This close relationship with the energy-releasing reactions and other body functions important to the athlete has prompted many to assume that vitamin supplements enhance performance—the "more is better" syndrome again! To help you educate your athletes about vitamins, let's look at what the research tells us.

Table 7.1
Vitamin Functions, Requirements, and Food Sources

Name of nutrient	Why you need it	How much do you need per day?	Daily needs met by:
Vitamin A	• To help keep skin smooth and soft • To help keep mucous membranes firm and resistant to infection • To protect against night blindness and promote healthy eyes	5,000 IU	Carrots—1 raw Spinach—½ c cooked Sweet potato—1 small baked Apricots—1 c canned Cantaloupe—½ melon Peach—2 medium Broccoli—2 stalks 1 c cooked Winter squash—1 c
The B Vitamins: Thiamine, riboflavin, and niacin	• To play a central role in the release of energy from food • To help the nervous system function properly • To help keep appetite and digestion normal • To help skin heal	Thiamine—1.5 mg	Needs partially (50%) met by: Lean pork—3 oz Lean beef, fish, and poultry—3 oz Bread, enriched—4 slices
		Riboflavin—1.7 mg	Milk, low-fat or skim—½ c Kidney beans—½ c canned Peas, green—½ c Green, leafy vegetables—½ c Lean ground beef—1 patty Baked salmon—3 oz
		Niacin—20 mg	Lean beef, pork, poultry, and fish Bread, enriched—1 slice Peanut butter—1 T

Vitamin	Functions	Amount	Food Sources
Vitamin B₆	• To help prevent anemia • Helps the body use and make protein	2.0 mg	Whole grains, vegetables, and meats
Vitamin B₁₂ and folacin	• To help enzyme and other biochemical systems function normally	Vitamin B₁₂—6 micrograms Folacin—0.4 mg	Lean beef, poultry, fish—4 oz Romaine lettuce—6 oz Spinach (cooked)—2 c
Vitamin C or ascorbic acid	• Helps hold body cells together and strengthens walls of blood vessels • To help resist infection • To help prevent fatigue • Aids in healing wounds and broken bones • Helps teeth and bone formation and promotes healthy gums • Helps body to absorb iron	60 mg	Citrus juice—6 oz Kiwi fruit—¼ whole Broccoli—½ stalk Brussels sprouts—4 Green pepper—1 Cantaloupe—½ Tomatoes—1½ medium
Vitamin D or the sunshine vitamin	• To help the body absorb calcium from digestive tract • To help build calcium and phosphorus into bones	400 IU	30 minutes of sunlight Fortified milk—4 c Salmon—3 oz
Vitamin E	• Helps with tissue growth, cell wall integrity, red blood cell integrity	30 IU	Green leafy vegetables—1½ lb Wheat germ—2 oz Vegetable oil—1 oz

FAT-SOLUBLE VITAMINS

Because they are not readily excreted from the body, the potential exists for a dangerous buildup of fat-soluble vitamins in the liver. In fact, there are case studies of athletes who overdosed on one or more of the fat-soluble vitamins, resulting in headaches, weight loss, and other symptoms that prevented them from being able to train. If the excessive consumption is not stopped, the damage to the body could even become life-threatening. Therefore, give special attention to educating your athletes about the dangers of supplementing these vitamins.

Vitamins A and D

Vitamin A is a label used to identify several components that, when converted to the active form, influence eyesight, the maintenance of skin and the mucous membranes, and the development of bones and teeth. The compounds labeled as *Vitamin D* also play a role in the development of bone. In spite of these vital functions, there is no research to support the use of vitamin A and D supplements by athletes (Williams, 1985). Instead, encourage athletes to obtain their vitamins A and D from a well-balanced diet. Liver and dairy products, including whole milk, margarine, and eggs, are the food sources with the highest quantities of vitamin A. These foods are also high in fat content. Because carbohydrates are the preferred fuel for athletes, encourage your athletes to use the high-carbohydrate foods listed in Table 7.1 as their sources for vitamin A, and discourage them from using vitamin A supplements. It is almost impossible to overdose on carrots, but vitamin A supplements could be very dangerous.

Although many high-fat foods, including liver, whole milk, and eggs, are also high in vitamin D, many other low-fat foods are artificially fortified with that vitamin. This factor, in combination with the fact that when we spend time outside in the sunlight, our bodies manufacture vitamin D, means that your athletes should have no trouble getting the required amount of vitamin D. Drinking fortified low-fat milk provides adequate vitamin D without running the risk of toxicity that can accompany vitamin D supplementation.

Vitamin E

At various times, proponents of vitamin E supplementation have claimed that this vitamin increases stamina, improves circulation and the delivery of oxygen to the muscles, lowers cholesterol, prevents graying hair, and cures infertility (Williams, 1985). Most of these claims are based on animal research findings. For example, some years ago, a group of researchers devised a vitamin E-deficient diet, which they fed to rats. Among the symptoms the rats exhibited was sterility. When vitamin E was returned to their diet, they became potent again (Pike & Brown, 1975). There is a great temptation to generalize these findings and say that vitamin E cures infertility in humans, but follow-up studies with humans have revealed that millions of people, especially athletes, who spend enormous sums of money on vitamin E capsules, solutions, fortifiers, skin lotions, and other products are doing so needlessly (Williams, 1985).

In answer to other claims, scientists have failed to verify that large supplements of vitamin E are in any way related to better athletic performance, although there is some research to support the claim that vitamin E may help to decrease the losses in aerobic endurance experienced at high altitude (Kobayashi, 1974). By eating nutritious foods, an individual can consume an optimal amount of vitamin E. Let your athletes know that vegetable oils, unrefined cereal products (especially those containing wheat germ), and eggs are good sources of vitamin E. White bread, junk food, and soda pop contain relatively little vitamin E.

At one time it was thought that vitamin E was nontoxic, but some findings indicate that overzealous supplementation (more than 2,000 IU per kilogram, which is 60 times the 30 IU per day requirement) may be harmful (National Research Council, 1974). To avoid such problems, encourage athletes to eat proper diets high in leafy vegetables and cereals (see Table 7.1) to obtain ample vitamin E.

Vitamin K

The *K* in vitamin K stands for the Danish word *koagulation*, which means coagulation or clotting. The vitamin has been so named because it is involved in the making of several proteins required for blood to clot. Although deficiencies are possible, they are rare in young athletes because vitamin K is made by the bacteria that live in the healthy intestine. In addition milk, green leafy vegetables, and some members of the cabbage family are excellent sources of vitamin K. While deficiencies are highly unlikely, vitamin K supplements can lead to toxicities. Therefore there is no need for athletes to take vitamin K supplements.

WATER-SOLUBLE VITAMINS

These vitamins are not typically stored in the body. Because they dissolve in water, excessive amounts of water-soluble vitamins are washed from the body, primarily in the urine. The B vitamins and vitamin C are the vitamins classified as water-soluble.

The B Vitamins

Included in the B complex are thiamine (B_1), riboflavin (B_2), niacin, pyridoxine (B_6), pantothenic acid, folic acid, cyanocobalamin (B_{12}), and biotin, but vitamins B_1, B_2, niacin, and B_6 have received the most research attention. As you can see in Table 7.1, the B vitamins are critical to the reactions that release energy. Therefore, they are of considerable interest to athletes and coaches. If an athlete has B complex deficiencies, endurance performance is impaired (Early & Carlson, 1969; Haymes, 1983) because endurance depends on sustained energy production. It is not surprising that in studies where individuals with B complex deficiencies were given B vitamin supplementation, the supplements were shown to be valuable. The influence of supplements on a diet that is already adequate is more controversial and needs more research.

Vitamins B_1 and B_2

Some of the research that has been conducted with thiamine (B_1) and riboflavin (B_2) suggests that athletes have greater requirements of these vitamins than nonathletes (Belko, et al., 1983; Colgan, 1982), although other studies have not verified these observations (Tremblay, Boilard, Breton, Bessette, & Roberge,

1984). Regardless of increased requirements, you should be aware that if your athletes eat a balanced diet by selecting high-carbohydrate, low-fat foods from the four basic food groups, they will more than meet the daily requirements for thiamine and riboflavin. For example, according to the four food group plan, a teenage athlete should consume three to four cups of low-fat milk, four servings of fruits and vegetables, two servings from the meat and meat substitutes group, and four servings from the grains (bread and cereal) category. If these servings are from foods like those listed in Table 7.1, the athlete will take in two to three times the daily requirements of thiamine and riboflavin.

An interesting paradox exists for many young athletes. Typically, they have heard that sugar is a quick energy source. So they happily stuff themselves with sugar-laden junk foods under the pretense that they are consuming quick energy. What these athletes fail to realize is that by eating candies and goodies instead of carbohydrates from fruits, vegetables, and grains, they are depriving themselves of needed B complex vitamins. Their vitamin B_1 requirement has increased because they are burning more energy while training, but the sugar in soda pop, candy, and other alleged quick energy sources contains no vitamin B_1.

Consumption of most sources of complex sugars or carbohydrates, such as fruits and vegetables, does not present this problem because those foods contain vitamin B_1 and other B complex vitamins. Athletes who fulfill their energy needs with junk foods run the risk of vitamin B_1 deficiency (Brin & Bauernfeind, 1978). In fact, this situation is becoming alarmingly common among teenagers in general. No athlete can hope to achieve his or her optimal performance capabilities under such conditions. You can help athletes by providing them with a well-thought-out nutritional conditioning program. A balanced diet is a much better approach to nutrition than encouraging youngsters to pop vitamin pills. Such a practice merely reinforces the belief that pills can solve all our problems.

Niacin

Another of the B complex vitamins is niacin. In addition to its role in carbohydrate metabolism, niacin is indispensable for fat and protein metabolism. A diet deficient in niacin is inappropriate for athletes. Such a deficiency is *not* likely if the individual eats the foods listed in Table 7.1. The increased caloric consumption that accompanies training and the consumption of lean meats and enriched breads will easily provide the 20 milligrams of niacin that are needed each day (Williams, 1985).

Supplementation is not only unnecessary, it may be counterproductive. Large doses of niacin (1200 milligrams 1 hour before exercise) have been shown to decrease fat utilization and decrease the amount of work performed (Pernow & Saltin, 1971).

Vitamin C

Vitamin C, or ascorbic acid, is another water-soluble vitamin that has received considerable attention recently. Because it has been suggested that doses of 10 to 100 times the amounts available in the most nutritious diet are effective in preventing or shortening the duration of the common cold, some people take large doses of vitamin C. Such supplementation is still controversial—some studies have failed to show that vitamin C has these effects on normal individuals.

Why should vitamin C alleviate cold symptoms? In test tubes, vitamin C detoxifies histamine, a product that is released in the body in response to various stresses (including the common cold). Although this occurs in the test tube, we are not sure of the extent to which it occurs in the living human.

It has been theorized that vitamin C supplementation can be valuable to athletes who constantly subject themselves to the stresses of physical training. Furthermore, ample evidence supports the important role of vitamin C in collagen synthesis (Williams, 1985). Collagen is an important constituent of the connective tissues of the body. The athlete in training is in constant need of collagen synthesis to strengthen existing connective tissue and to develop new tissue.

In light of these biological contributions and because vitamin C is a water-soluble vitamin and toxicities from large doses have been thought to be unlikely, many people have advocated vitamin C supplementation for athletes. There is little research to support such a suggestion, however (Haymes, 1983).

Furthermore, there are an increasing number of problems reported to be associated with taking large doses of vitamin C (Whitney & Hamilton, 1981). Once again, the preferred method for increasing vitamin consumption is eating a balanced diet consisting of greater quantities of fruits, vegetables, and whole grains. For example, 6 ounces of orange juice and half a stalk of broccoli provides twice the amount of vitamin C that is needed per day (see Table 7.1).

THE BALANCED DIET

The critical issue is the ease with which an athlete who is training hard can eat a well-balanced diet. A balanced diet is defined as one that includes

- dairy foods such as milk, cheese, and yogurt;
- fruits and vegetables, especially yellow and leafy green vegetables, as well as oranges, grapefruit, or raw green peppers;
- whole-grain or enriched bread, cereal, macaroni, spaghetti, or rice; and
- high-protein food such as meat, fish, poultry, soybeans, and legumes.

This four food group approach to a balanced diet, which was introduced in chapter 3, works even though the athlete's increased caloric expenditure may increase the need for some of the water-soluble vitamins. For example, as previously mentioned, the requirement for vitamin B_1 or thiamine increases with energy expenditure (National Research Council, 1974). Therefore, the more calories burned, as in training, the greater the body's need for thiamine. This increased need can be easily met by the four food group plan as long as athletes select foods that are high in nutrient content. If athletes choose empty calorie foods, which have energy value but few vitamins and minerals, they may obtain less-than-optimal amounts of nutrient.

ADDITIONAL FACTORS IN VITAMIN ABSORPTION

In working with the four food groups to prepare a balanced diet, athletes should be aware of some factors that influence vitamin absorption. Keep these factors in mind as you assist your athletes in refining their nutrition plans.

Vitamin Loss in Sweat

In addition to their increased energy use as a result of training, athletes also lose a considerable amount of body water as sweat. Because the B complex vitamins and vitamin C dissolve in water, increased sweat loss means an increased loss of vitamins. Vitamins lost in this manner can be replaced, but only if the athlete makes wise food choices. Without careful selection, these vitamins may not be replaced in the system.

The Dieting Athlete

If an athlete is on a diet to lose weight, the increased need for vitamin B_1 associated with increased energy expenditure and the vitamin losses due to increased sweating may not be met. Therefore some supplementation has been suggested for athletes who are restricting their caloric intake (Williams, 1985). A good multiple vitamin is the best approach, because it contains all the vitamins, a situation that more closely approximates eating food.

Aspirin

If an athlete routinely takes aspirin for an injury, deficits in iron, vitamin C, and folacin (one of the B complex vitamins) may occur. Aspirin decreases the absorption of these substances (Whitney & Hamilton, 1981). An athlete who eats nutritious foods can obtain the increased amount of needed nutrient without supplementation.

SUMMARY AND RECOMMENDATIONS

We have repeatedly emphasized that taking separate pills for each vitamin does not make good nutritional sense. Optimal body function does not depend just on taking in vitamins; these vitamins must be available in the right combinations and quantities. This is why we advocate *eating* the food sources of these vitamins rather than "pill popping" as the foundation for nutritional conditioning. Furthermore, advocating the use of vitamin pills can result in athletes adopting unrealistic expectations about the pills, causing athletes to neglect their rest, eating, and training habits. Foods, with their naturally available vitamins and nutrients, are the best way of meeting the body's needs as well as assuring that vitamin overdoses do not occur.

The possible exception to this emphasis on food is the smaller, lighter athlete or one involved in weight reduction. Dietary vitamin supplements can help these athletes meet their nutrient requirements on a restricted caloric intake.

To help athletes learn to make wise food choices that ensure adequate vitamin consumption, you should take the following steps:

1. Introduce the four food group plan to your athletes and their parents.
2. Provide athletes and parents with practical information relative to the implementation of the four food group plan as a strategy for eating a high-carbohydrate, low-fat diet. For example, sample meal plans such as those listed in chapter 14 could help. In addition, there are a number of high-carbohydrate, low-fat cookbooks in print. Look for them at your local bookstore.
3. Work to have high-carbohydrate, low-fat snack food choices available to your athletes. For example, when food is sold at athletic events, be sure that cold, crisp, fresh fruits are available for purchase and that the choices are not limited to high-fat potato chips and chocolate candy bars. In your organization, can athletes purchase fruit juices, or are no-nutrient soda pops the only drinks sold? Are low-fat sandwiches on the menu, or are only hot dogs and other high-fat sandwiches available?
4. Suggest that athletes who are restricting their caloric intake and who therefore may be in jeopardy of developing vitamin deficiencies take a multiple vitamin preparation.

Chapter 8
Minerals

Minerals are the inorganic substances of the body. The body needs many minerals, including sodium, chloride, calcium, phosphorus, magnesium, sulfur, and at least 14 trace minerals. A detailed discussion of sodium, potassium, and chloride, commonly called electrolytes, is presented in chapter 10. The minerals associated with bone metabolism—calcium, phosphorus, and magnesium—as well as iron and zinc are discussed in this chapter.

BONE MINERALS

Bones and teeth are made of both organic materials and inorganic minerals, including calcium, phosphorus, and magnesium.

Calcium

Calcium is the most abundant of the three. In general it accounts for about 1.5% to 2% of an adult's total body weight. Although 99% of the calcium is in the bones and teeth, the remaining 1% is also very important; it plays a vital role in the contraction of muscles, the transmission of nerve impulses, the functioning of cell membranes, the clotting processes, and the breakdown of glycogen (Williams, 1985).

The concept of calcium balance is based on the notion that the dietary calcium absorbed must equal the calcium lost from the body. The amount of calcium to be consumed consequently sounds like an easy fact to determine. In reality it is quite complicated.

Growth is a major complicating variable. The skeleton increases in size and density during the growth years and requires increased calcium, as reflected by the suggested calcium intake values presented in Table 8.1.

Table 8.1
Recommended Dietary Allowances for Calcium for Normal, Healthy Individuals

Age	mg/day[1] (RDA)	mg/day[2]
0-0.5 yr	360	
0.5-1.0 yr	540	
1-10 yr	800	
10-18 yr	1,200	
Premenopausal	800	1,000-1,200
Postmenopausal	800	1,200-1,500

[1]National Research Council, 1980.
[2]Avioli, 1987.

If adequate calcium is not taken in and absorbed during the period of growth and after peak bone mass is achieved, the individual will be in negative calcium balance. The word *absorbed* used here is a key term. Not all of the calcium that enters the body in food is absorbed.

Growth and absorption, then, complicate the process of achieving calcium balance. Because of these complications, many authorities believe that the RDA values should be increased for both pre- and postmenopausal women (Avioli, 1987). These specific increases are presented in Table 8.1.

Skeletal Growth

Unfortunately, most people believe that skeletal growth refers only to the long growth of bones, a process that ends at about age 20 (National Dairy Council, 1984). Few realize that the bones continue to grow in density and thickness until 30 to 40 years of age. After that time bone density is gradually lost as a function of aging. If an individual has a lower peak bone mass, it will take fewer years of age-related losses of bone density to result in osteoporosis and an increased risk of fractures.

Women have a lower peak bone mass than males and therefore are more likely to suffer from osteoporosis. Whether calcium consumption during a person's lifetime can influence the rate of osteoporosis development is somewhat controversial, but there is a growing body of information to support the concept that calcium intake is important in this regard (Avioli, 1987). Therefore it is critical that all females take special precautions to ensure adequate calcium absorption so that they can achieve their true peak bone mass. This precautionary step may be even more important for females who are athletes.

Calcium Absorption

Athletes who wish to get adequate amounts of calcium should be aware of foods that are sources of calcium as well as factors that influence calcium absorption. A typical list of calcium food sources is presented in Table 8.2. A list like this provides little indication as to how much of the calcium will actually be absorbed. The absorption of calcium from dairy products is quite good, but the absorption of calcium from plant foods is quite poor (Allen, 1984). Apparently fiber and other substances in plants impair calcium absorption. If a person's diet contains only a small amount of calcium, calcium absorption will increase, but there is a limit to the effectiveness of this process over time. If too little calcium is ingested for too long a period, bone density will not be optimal.

Calcium Deficiency

In an individual with a calcium deficiency, bone density will not be as great, leading to osteoporosis. Because females have a smaller bone mass than males and because the availability of the female hormone estrogen, which influences bone density, decreases after menopause, osteoporosis is more common among women, particularly older women, than among men.

Coaches of young women should be concerned about their athletes' bone health for several reasons. Osteoporotic bone is more

susceptible to fracture than normal bone (Heaney, 1987). Dunn (1981) and others have hypothesized that low calcium intake could be the reason that ballet dancers experience an increased incidence of stress fractures. Other groups of female performers who routinely diet, including distance runners and gymnasts, also experience a relatively high rate of stress fractures (Nilson, 1986). Loss of calcium from the body may also contribute to muscle cramps (Williams, 1985).

A number of surveys conducted by various governmental agencies—for example the Ten-State Nutrition Survey (U.S. Department of Health, Education, and Welfare, 1972) and the HANES I survey (U.S. Department of Health, Education, and Welfare, 1974)—report that most females do not consume the RDA values for calcium. Furthermore, the HANES I survey demonstrated that 6% to 18% of the females between 25 and 34 years of age had decreased bone mass.

Based on the dietary survey information about female athletes, particularly those involved in sports and activities that require weight control such as distance running, gymnastics, figure skating, and ballet, many of these women are like their sedentary counterparts in that they consume inadequate amounts of calcium (Drinkwater et al., 1984; Dunn, 1981). The long-term consequences of weight-watching female athletes' low calcium intakes have yet to be documented, but given the incidence of decreased bone density observed in the HANES I survey, many have speculated that low dietary intake places an athlete at increased risk for low bone density. Although the mechanical stresses associated with physical activity are known to have a positive effect on bone density (Avioli, 1987), if the body suffers from inadequate dietary calcium, the positive effects of exercise may not be fully realized.

Reduced calcium intake has even more dramatic effects in amenorrheic athletes. Several researchers have observed that female athletes who are amenorrheic (i.e., those whose menstrual periods have been suppressed, sometimes as a result of intense physical exertion) have lower bone density in their vertebrae than athletes who are menstruating normally (Cann, Martin, Genant, & Jaffe, 1984; Drinkwater et al., 1984). This may involve a decrease in estrogen in the amenorrheic athlete. Estrogen plays an important role in the maintenance of bone density (Heaney, 1987). More research is needed on this topic and how increased calcium intake may change bone density readings.

Because of their relatively larger body size and caloric intake, relatively few male athletes or their sedentary counterparts are calcium-deficient. Though it is true that an increase in protein consumption may increase calcium excretion in the urine, male athletes typically have enough calcium in their diets to compensate for this loss. Similarly, even though increased amounts of calcium can be lost in sweat, the dietary intake of most male athletes is sufficient to maintain adequate calcium balance.

Increased Calcium Intake

Calcium is a major constituent of bone; bones that have a low density or are osteoporotic have a lower calcium content. The role of increased calcium intake as a strategy for preventing osteoporosis is an interesting topic. Many coaches wonder if increased calcium consumption helps to increase vertebral bone density in amenorrheic athletes. One recent study suggests that additional calcium will not completely restore bone density in this instance. Again, much more research is needed on this topic, but at this point we suggest that female athletes pay particular attention to eating high-calcium foods (see Table 8.2). Amenorrheic athletes should consult with their physicians about increasing their daily calcium consumption above 1,000 milligrams per day. Though it appears that calcium deficiency can impair an athlete's potential for physical performance by altering the normal function of the neuromuscular system and the breakdown of glycogen as well as increasing the risk of stress fractures, it should also be noted that excessive calcium intake may result in kidney stone formation, particularly in individuals with a family history of such problems.

Phosphorus

Phosphorus is another mineral found in bones and teeth. It is also involved in the energy-releasing chemical reactions in the body and is part of the high-energy compounds ATP (adenosine triphosphate) and PC (phosphocreatine). Phosphorus is found in many foods (see Table 8.2), and consequently deficiencies do not seem to be a problem. Though some researchers believe that increased phosphorus consumption increases calcium excretion, this does not seem to be a problem unless very extreme amounts are consumed (Avioli, 1987). Such extremes are not likely unless an individual takes phosphorus supplements.

Magnesium

Magnesium is a mineral involved in a number of the body's functions—energy metabolism, nerve impulse transmission, muscle contraction, and protein synthesis. It is readily available in a number of foods (see Table 8.2) and therefore magnesium deficiencies rarely occur. There are, however, accounts of individuals who after prolonged bouts of diarrhea or profuse sweat loss experienced weakness and muscle cramps as a result of magnesium deficiencies (Williams, 1985). Because excessive magnesium in the diet can cause diarrhea, athletes should replenish magnesium lost in the sweat with foods that contain magnesium rather than with supplements to avoid overdoses.

IRON

Advertisements warning of "iron-poor blood" are familiar to many Americans, but these ads usually feature middle-aged women rather than athletes. Recently, some case histories have highlighted the iron needs of athletes, particularly those involved in endurance sports.

In 1984, Alberto Salazar, the world's fastest marathon runner, was neither sleeping nor performing well. A blood test proved he was iron-deficient, and his physician prescribed iron supplementation. In the following weeks he began sleeping better and his performance improved.

As athletes and coaches heard of Salazar's experience, there was a surge of interest in iron-deficiency anemia, blood testing, and iron supplementation. As a result of this emphasis on iron, many athletes adopted iron supplementation programs whether their bodies

Table 8.2

Mineral Functions, Requirements, and Food Sources

Name of nutrient	Why you need it	How much do you need per day?	Daily needs met by:
Calcium	• To help build bones, teeth • To help blood clot • To help muscles contract and relax normally • To delay fatigue and help tired muscles recover	1,000 mg	Milk or yogurt—4 c Cheese—3½ oz Broccoli, mustard greens—2½ c
Phosphorus	• To build bones • To make the energy molecule ATP • To utilize glucose as fuel	800 mg	Roast turkey or fish—6 oz Skim milk—3 oz Roast chicken—7 oz
Magnesium	• To help regulate the heart and skeletal muscles • To obtain energy from the fuel foods	350 mg	Whole-grain cereal—3 c Legumes—3 c Dark green vegetables—3 c cooked
Iron	• To make hemoglobin in red blood cells that carries oxygen to the cells of the body	10 mg (men) 18 mg (women)	Needs partially (50%) met by: Beef, lamb, pork—6 oz Baked beans—2 c Prunes—18 Chicken, fish—8 oz
Zinc	• To help normal cell division, tissue growth, and injury repair	15 mg	Crab meat—9 oz Turkey—9 oz Wheat germ—3 oz Garbanzo beans—3½ c
Chromium	• To maintain normal blood glucose levels • To aid protein synthesis	50-100 mg	Potatoes with skin—4 large Oysters—3 Wheat germ—¾ c Wheat bran—1 c

needed them or not. In addition to being expensive, iron supplementation is potentially dangerous because excess iron cannot be eliminated from the body and is stored in the liver. Permanent liver damage may occur in an individual who consumes too much iron (White, Handler, & Smith, 1973).

Iron is an important constituent of hemoglobin (the substance that transports 98% of the oxygen in the blood), myoglobin (the substance that helps transport oxygen within muscle cells), and the cytochromes (substances required for the aerobic burning of fuels). Endurance athletes must be capable of transporting large quantities of oxygen to cells, and the aerobic machinery in the cells must be capable of using this oxygen to burn the fuel foods. Because of all this, iron is important to the endurance athlete for both circulatory and metabolic reasons. If anemic individuals take iron supplements, maximum oxygen capacity and the ability to do physical work are enhanced (Gardner, Edgerton, Senewiratne, Baranard, & Ohira, 1977). However, determination of anemia and the optimal doses for iron supplementation give rise to many controversies.

Terminology

To better understand the issues surrounding iron status and the athlete, we will first examine some of the terminology used in literature. *Anemia* refers to the situation where an individual has a reduced amount of hemoglobin in the blood. The normal range of hemoglobin for males is 14 to 18 grams per deciliter (g/dl) of blood, which is higher than the normal range for women (12 to 16 g/dl). Typically males with hemoglobin values below 14 g/dl and females with values below 12 g/dl are classified as anemic (Wintrobe, 1981). If the anemia is due to inadequate availability of iron for making hemoglobin, the term *iron-deficiency anemia* is used.

The observation that the hemoglobin levels of many endurance athletes are lower than the mean values for sedentary men and women (16 g/dl and 14 g/dl, respectively), prompted the term *sports anemia* (Pate, 1983). However, this term is a misuse of the word anemia according to one researcher (Eichner, 1986). Just because hemoglobin values are at the lower end of the normal range (14 to 16 g/dl

for men and 12 to 14 g/dl for women) does not mean that an athlete is anemic. Anemia has been defined by specific values. To be consistent, the term sports anemia should not be used to describe athletes with hemoglobin values that are merely in the lower range for their gender.

As a result Pate (1983) and others have suggested a new term for describing the situation where an athlete's hemoglobin values are in the lower end of the normal range. The term *suboptimal hemoglobin* points out that although hemoglobin levels in the lower normal range do not indicate anemia, they may prevent the athlete from attaining optimal endurance performance. Therefore a male's hemoglobin level of between 14 and 16 g/dl is thought to be a suboptimal level for performance, and the suboptimal hemoglobin level for females is thought to be between 12 and 14 g/dl (Pate, 1983).

Iron Deficiency Stages

In the past, evaluation of hemoglobin concentration has typically been used to screen for anemia. It may not actually be the best tool, however. Hemoglobin may be the last entity affected by iron deficiency (Plowman & McSwegin, 1981). Sport scientists have suggested that there are stages of iron deficiency that appear prior to the occurrence of anemia, and these should be evaluated in athletes. To better understand these stages, let us first examine how iron is absorbed and used.

Iron that is absorbed from the intestine (the factors that influence absorption are discussed later) is transported in the serum of the blood by a protein carrier called *transferrin*. Transferrin also transports iron saved from red blood cells (RBC) that have been destroyed and iron that is being taken from the liver to tissues that require iron. With this system, bone marrow (where hemoglobin-containing RBCs are made) and other tissues that need iron can receive it. In an individual with suboptimal iron consumption, inadequate amounts of iron are available for storage. Due to the low iron storage levels, less iron will be available for transit. These decreases in stored and transit iron will eventually result in decreased blood hemoglobin levels.

Measurement of stored iron, iron in transit, and hemoglobin provide a more comprehensive picture of the body's iron status than measurement of hemoglobin alone. For example, the material in Table 8.3 illustrates that a hemoglobin value of 14 g/dl can occur even if the amount of iron in storage and in transport is deficient. In other words, decreased iron consumption and absorption decrease the amount of iron in transit as well as the amount in storage. But these decreases do not immediately decrease hemoglobin levels. Whether such decreases in storage iron decrease the iron provided to the cytochromes and other substances required for aerobic metabolism is controversial. Some researchers (Clements & Sawchuk, 1984) say that they do and others (Eichner, 1986) disagree. Furthermore, several studies in which iron supplements were given to athletes with suboptimal but not anemic levels of hemoglobin failed to demonstrate significant improvements in iron status (Pate, Maguire, & Van Wyk, 1979) or in performance. Sport scientists have therefore been hesitant to suggest that all endurance athletes should consume more than the RDA for iron or take iron supplements.

Causes of Suboptimal Hemoglobin Concentrations

Perhaps the reason for the inconsistencies in the research discussed above is the fact that normal hemoglobin and iron status indicators vary from individual to individual. In addition, a number of things can cause suboptimal hemoglobin concentrations.

Dilution Effect

Many athletes respond to training by retaining sodium, which results in an increase in the volume of water in the blood (Williams, 1985). This expanded plasma volume could serve to dilute the blood, explaining reduced hemoglobin concentration. Not all athletes, however, experience such a change in plasma volume (Scheur & Tipton, 1977), and not all of the changes seen in blood variables can be accounted for by a simple dilution effect (Puhl et al., 1985).

RBC Destruction

Another explanation for the somewhat low hemoglobin levels seen in many athletes is that these athletes are experiencing a high rate of red blood cell (RBC) destruction. Typically, red blood cells survive in the blood for about 120 days. As a result, we lose about 1% of our RBCs every day. If all of the iron in these cells were lost it would represent about 25 milligrams of iron; fortunately much of this iron is usually recaptured and reused. In runners, however, it has been suggested that the impact of the foot striking the ground increases

Table 8.3
Stages of Iron Deficiency

Stage	Measure of storage iron Ferritin (mg/L)	Measure of transport iron % Sat[1]	Measure of anemia HB (g/dl)
Good	60	35	14
Suboptimal	20	35	14
Deficient	12	16	13
Anemia	12	16	12

Note. From "Iron Status and Training" by J.L. Puhl, P.J. Van Handel, L.L. Williams, P.W. Bradley, and S.J. Harms. In *The Elite Athlete* (p. 217) by N.K. Butts, T.T. Gushiken, and B. Zarins, (Eds.), 1985, Champaign, IL: Life Enhancement Publications. Copyright 1985 by Nancy K. Butts, Thomas T. Gushiken, and Bertram Zarins. Modified by permission.

[1]% Sat = percentage of the iron carrier transferrin that is saturated with iron.

the destruction of RBCs (also called hemolysis). Because of the increased rate of destruction, more iron than normal is lost, and the body's iron stores may be depleted (Eichner, 1986). This footstrike hemolysis is one of the reasons that blood may appear in the urine following an arduous training session.

Blood Loss in the Gastrointestinal Tract

Another explanation for suboptimal hemoglobin concentrations, iron deficiency, or both among some groups of athletes stems from the observation that many runners lose a substantial amount of blood into the gastrointestinal tract (Stewart, Ahlquist, McGill, Ilstrup, Schwartz, & Owen, 1984). The reason for this blood loss is not fully understood; however, the added stresses inherent in running are considered possible explanations.

Iron Losses in Sweat

One of the constituents of sweat is iron. Therefore, increased quantities of sweat lost with increased levels of training may increase the likelihood of an iron deficiency.

Inadequate Intake

The individual who is not eating a balanced diet and does not take in a sufficient number of calories may not be replacing iron losses. Such a diet might also be lacking in vitamin C (necessary for iron absorption), protein, vitamin B_{12}, or folic acid, all of which are needed to make RBCs. Therefore, dietary deficiency may be a cause of suboptimal hemoglobin concentration or iron deficiency.

Suboptimal Hemoglobin Risk Groups

Ideally there should be a daily balance between the iron absorbed and the iron lost. For example, typical American diets contain about 6 milligrams (mg) of iron per 1,000 kilocalories (kcal). The quantity of iron that the body actually absorbs is variable and usually ranges between 5% and 35%. So an athlete who consumes 2,000 kcal a day gets about 12 mg of iron, and 0.6 to 4.2 mg is absorbed. For nonexercising men and women, normal daily iron losses have been determined to be 0.9 mg per

day for men and 1.5 mg per day for women. (The higher value for women reflects menstrual blood losses.) According to these calculations, individuals whose bodies have good absorption of iron (closer to 35% than to 5%), who consume at least 2,000 kcal per day, and who are not losing too much iron are not at risk for iron deficiencies.

However, individuals who eat fewer than 2,000 kcal per day or who are losing iron as a result of footstrike hemolysis, heavy sweat, or blood loss in the gastrointestinal tract are at risk for iron deficiencies. This means that male endurance athletes, adolescent male athletes, most female athletes, and any athlete who restricts caloric intake may be at risk for iron deficiency. The adolescent male athlete is somewhat vulnerable because he needs iron during his growth spurt (Feinstein & Daniel, 1984). Women in general are at risk because the average adult woman loses about 40 to 45 milliliters of blood each menstrual period, totaling about 14 to 15 mg of iron per cycle. With other iron losses 1.4 to 1.5 mg of iron are lost per day (Puhl et al., 1985). Therefore adult females have a higher daily iron requirement than do adult males: an RDA of 18 mg per day. As stated previously, the typical American diet contains about 6 mg of iron per 1,000 kcal. An individual with low (10%) iron absorption has to ingest about 2,514 kcal to obtain the required iron. If iron absorption is very high (30%), only about 1,200 kcal needs to be ingested (Puhl et al., 1985). In reality a 30% rate of absorption is rare, and typically, women eat less than 2,500 kcal per day; therefore, women frequently have lower iron intakes than are recommended.

Female athletes who participate in sports such as distance running, gymnastics, and figure skating have an even higher risk of iron deficiency because they are likely to be restricting caloric intake. The risk is even greater if these women eat foods low in iron and do not take steps to maximize iron absorption.

Maximizing Iron Absorption

One of the factors that influences iron absorption is the type of iron ingested. *Heme iron*, which makes up 50% to 60% of the iron in beef, lamb, and chicken and about 30% to 40% of the iron in fish, liver, and pork, is absorbed at a rate of 15% to 35%. The absorption rate is closer to 35% if the body's iron stores are low (Puhl et al., 1985). It is estimated that 23% of dietary heme iron is absorbed. *Non-heme iron* accounts for the rest of the iron found in meats and all of the iron in fruits, vegetables, dried beans, nuts, and grain products. Non-heme iron is not absorbed as readily as heme iron and is more dependent upon the other constituents of the meal. Some good sources of iron are listed in Tables 8.2 and 8.4.

Table 8.4
Iron Content of Some Common Foods

Source	Quantity	Iron (mg)
Heme Iron		
Calf liver	3.5 oz	9
Lean steak	3.5 oz	4.5
Pork chop	3.5 oz	4.5
Lamb	3.5 oz	3
Turkey, dark meat	3.5 oz	2.5
Chicken, dark meat	3.5 oz	2
Tuna	3.5 oz	2
Chicken, light meat	3.5 oz	1
Turkey, light meat	3.5 oz	1
Salmon	3.5 oz	1
Non-Heme Iron		
Dried apricots	12	6
Prune juice	½ c	5
Dates	9	5
Baked beans	½ c	3
Kidney beans	½ c	3
Molasses, blackstrap	1 T	3
Raisins	½ c	2
Spinach[1]	½ c	2
Tofu[2]	½ c	2
Brewer's yeast	1 T	2
Egg	1 medium	1
Enriched bread	1 slice	1
Enriched pasta	½ c	1
Peas, green	½ c	1
Molasses, regular	1 T	1
Wheat germ	1 T	1
Cheddar cheese	1 oz	trace
Peanut butter	1 oz	.5

[1]Spinach is high in phytates and therefore iron is not very available.

[2]The iron in tofu is quite absorbable even though it is a non-heme iron source.

An individual can enhance the absorption of non-heme iron by eating foods that contain vitamin C along with the non-heme iron sources (Rossander, Hallberg, & Bjorn-Rasmussen, 1979) and combining heme and non-heme iron sources, as in meat-and-vegetable casseroles, chili with beans, chicken tacos with beans, split-pea soup with ham, and turkey soup with lentils (Clark, 1985). Breakfast is a good opportunity to increase iron consumption. A bowl of Total cereal with skim milk and a small glass of orange juice provides more than 100% of the daily requirement for iron. Table 8.5 lists the iron content of other popular cereals.

Athletes should also be aware that the tannic acid in tea and high amounts of fiber and phytates (found in many vegetables) in the diet reduce iron absorption. Others have indicated that consumption of high quantities of caffeine also inhibits iron absorption.

Table 8.5
Iron Content of Some Breakfast Cereals

Cereal name	Iron (% RDA)
Total	100
Kellogg's 40% Bran Flakes	100
All-natural granola	45
Life	35
Cheerios	25
Wheat Chex	25
Post Raisin Bran	25
Captain Crunch	25
Quaker Instant Otameal	25
All-Bran	25
Corn flakes	10
Kellogg's Raisin Squares	10
Rice Crispies	10
Frosted Flakes	10
Shredded Wheat (mini)	4
Nutri-Grain	4
Grape-Nuts	4
Quaker 100% Natural	4
Puffed wheat	trace

ZINC, CHROMIUM, AND TRACE MINERALS

Knowledge about the athlete's need for zinc, chromium, and many of the other trace minerals (i.e., those that are present in the body only in minute amounts) is incomplete. Although it has been established that athletes experience greater zinc and chromium losses than do nonathletes (Anderson, Polansky, Bryden, & Guttman, 1986), it appears that wise food selections and a diet that does not restrict calories should be adequate to replace lost trace minerals (Dressendorfer, Wade, Keen, & Scatf, 1982). Some suggested food sources for zinc and chromium are listed in Table 8.2.

SUMMARY AND RECOMMENDATIONS

Minerals are important to the optimal functioning of the human body, and therefore coaches should encourage their athletes to consume adequate amounts of the minerals described in this chapter as well as those discussed in chapter 10. To accomplish the goal of optimal mineral consumption, you should take the following steps:

1. Encourage your athletes to select high-carbohydrate, low-fat foods from the four basic food groups.
2. Recognize that lightweight female athletes, especially if amenorrheic, may be at risk for calcium deficiency. It is particularly important for coaches to encourage these athletes to eat foods rich in calcium. Because small increases in calcium intake are not likely to be dangerous, a goal of 1,000 to 1,200 milligrams of calcium per day for premenopausal athletes and 1,200 to 1,500 milligrams per day for postmenopausal and amenorrheic athletes are appropriate goals. If food alone does not provide these quantities of calcium, supplementation is in order.
3. Select supplements wisely. Calcium carbonate supplements have the highest percentage of calcium but depend on acid in the stomach for absorption. Bone meal and dolomite should be avoided because of the possibility of lead poisoning. The antacid Tums contains calcium carbonate (200 milligrams per tablet) and can serve as a calcium supplement. Aluminum-containing antacids, however, should be avoided (Avioli, 1987). Certain medications also impair calcium absorption, so have your athletes check with their physicians before beginning supplementation.
4. Take steps to help insure that your athletes have optimal iron status. Inform them about foods that are particularly rich sources of heme iron but are low in fats. Also, cooking in iron pots increases the amount of iron in the diet. For example, the iron content of 1/2 cup of spaghetti sauce may increase from 3 to 88 milligrams if the sauce simmers in a cast-iron pot for 3 hours (Clark, 1985).
5. Encourage athletes, particularly females, who are restricting calories to give special attention to optimizing their intake of vitamin C, vitamin B_{12}, and folic acid as well as iron.
6. Discourage the indiscriminate use of iron supplements. Before an athlete begins to take iron supplements, blood tests to evaluate iron status should be administered. Such tests are most meaningful if they are administered three or four times a year so that changes for a given individual may be noted (Puhl et al., 1985). More research is needed before the optimal doses for iron supplementation are known, so consultation with a good sport medicine physician is essential.
7. Advocate the consumption of nutritious food rather than pills and supplements. If athletes or their parents press for some supplement suggestions, a good multiple vitamin, that contains iron (ferrous sulfate) is appropriate. However, avoid indiscriminate use of iron supplements, because too much iron in the body can lead to toxicity.

Chapter 9
Water, Water, Everywhere

Water is just as important to good nutrition as carbohydrates, fats, proteins, vitamins, and minerals are. Unfortunately, many athletes do not realize this—they restrict their water intake and use water loss to lose weight rapidly. You and your athletes must understand that water is vital during performance. In addition, you must also be aware of the circumstances that influence the body's water content. This chapter tells you about water—what it is, what it does, and why it is so important.

Water is a simple compound made up of two hydrogen atoms and one oxygen atom, as shown in the formula H_2O. It is essential not only for optimal physical performance, but for life itself. In a sport such as wrestling, athletes are sometimes more concerned about "making weight" than about how valuable water is to their performance. Because water weighs about 1 pound per pint, the body's weight can be reduced dramatically by limiting fluid consumption and stimulating water losses. The ramifications of water restriction, however, can be severe.

A healthy youngster's weight is 45% to 65% water. This is a larger value than for adults (Lohman, 1986). Although these percentages may sound high, none of this water represents excess. To explain why, let's examine where this water is located and how it contributes to life processes.

WATER COMPARTMENTS

Water is distributed in a number of different compartments or spaces within the body (see Figure 9.1). The extracellular compartment consists of all of those "spaces" in the body

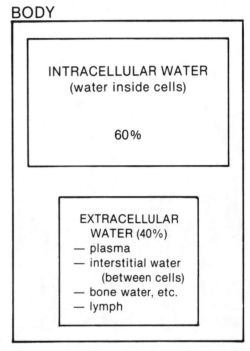

BODY

INTRACELLULAR WATER
(water inside cells)

60%

EXTRACELLULAR
WATER (40%)
— plasma
— interstitial water
    (between cells)
— bone water, etc.
— lymph

Figure 9.1. The body has two major water compartments. The intracellular compartment represents water held inside the cells of the body, whereas the extracellular compartment represents water found outside cells in such places as blood plasma, lymph, and cerebral spinal fluid.

that are located outside the cells and that contain water. Blood plasma, for instance, which is made up primarily of water, represents one of the extracellular spaces and constitutes about 5% of the body's weight. Extracellular water is also found in hollow organs like the eye, in the joints, and in bones, but the greatest quantity of extracellular fluid—the intercellular or interstitial fluid—surrounds and bathes the cells.

A larger amount of water is located *inside* the body's cells. This is known as intracellular fluid. The muscle cells in particular contain a great deal of water—so much of it, in fact, that over 70% of their weight is from water. Fat contains much less water. In addition, glucose is stored with water as glycogen (1 gram of glycogen to 2 grams of water) in the muscles. The trained athlete, on the left in Figure 9.2, has more stored glycogen than the untrained individual on the right. Consequently, he is leaner and has more body water than his nonathletic classmate, who has more body fat and less muscle glycogen. This does *not* mean, however, that the trained athlete can afford to lose more water weight.

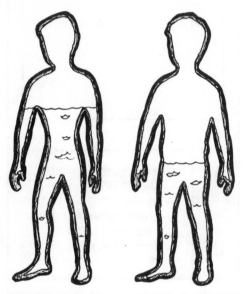

Figure 9.2. Muscle cells contain more water than do fat cells; therefore, the individual with more body fat has less body water than a well-conditioned athlete has.

WATER IS ESSENTIAL

Participants in high-energy-output and endurance activities especially need adequate levels of body water. For example, a Swiss team's unsuccessful attempt to climb Mount Everest was attributed to their small supply of water (see Figure 9.3). They had brought only enough fuel to melt snow for 1 pint of water per day per climber during their ascent. As the climbers became dehydrated, fatigue forced them to turn back. A later climbing party was successful, but they carried enough fuel to pro-

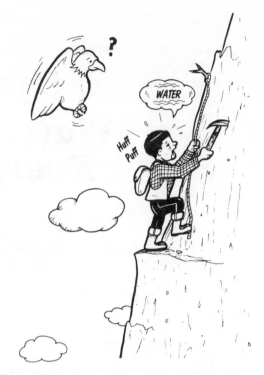

Figure 9.3. Adequate water is essential to preventing fatigue and allowing optimal muscular function.

vide each climber with 7 pints of water per day!

The athlete's need for body water can best be understood by briefly examining the functions of water in the body. Three functions are especially critical for physical activity.

Water as a Solvent

Because water is a medium compatible with many compounds, it serves as an excellent means of transporting substances. For example, various nutrients, hormones, and even antibodies are transported in the water of the blood plasma to the intercellular fluid, the water that surrounds the individual cells. Likewise, the waste products released by the cells are carried away by water. Without such a highly efficient transport mechanism, nourishment of the cells would be impossible.

Water as a Temperature Regulator

Water has two major roles to play in the process of regulating the body's temperature. First of all, water can absorb a considerable amount of heat before its temperature rises. Even while at rest, each of the cells of the body is continually burning fuels to provide energy for life processes. A large portion of the released energy is not useful energy; rather, it is heat energy (see Figure 9.4). This heat energy enables the individual to maintain a normal body temperature of about 98.6° Fahrenheit (37° centigrade). However, the excess heat must be dissipated so body temperature does not rise. The body's water serves that purpose. During physical activity, the body's energy need increases, and the rate at which fuel is burned increases accordingly. Under these circumstances, cooling procedures become even more important.

The cells of the body are similar to combustion engines in cars. As engines burn gasoline, energy is given off as heat. An automobile has a cooling system to prevent the engine from overheating. Similarly, if the heat given off by the muscle cells and the other cells of the body is not dispelled from the body, the body temperature soars, destroying structural proteins as well as the enzymes that regulate the various chemical reactions in the body.

Because each tissue is made up of thousands of layers of cells, dissipating the heat directly into the environment would be too slow a process. Instead, the intercellular water that surrounds the cells and makes up the circulating blood plasma works much like the water cooling system that cools your car's engine. The plasma picks up the heat and carries it to the skin's surface, where the heat escapes into the environment. If the heart did not continually pump blood to circulate the plasma, enabling it to absorb heat from the cells, and if

water could not absorb such large quantities of heat so readily, it would be very difficult for the body to cool itself.

This ingenious cooling system is able to work efficiently only if blood volume and intercellular fluid volume are adequate. Just as the car's engine will overheat if the water level in the radiator is too low, the body's cooling system will also fail if the volume of circulating water (blood and intercellular fluid) is decreased. This is exactly what happens when athletes choose to lose weight by getting rid of water or dehydrating. Sweating in steam rooms, using diuretic pills, and engaging in any other procedures that result in the rapid loss of 2% or more of a person's body weight due to dehydration result in reduced efficiency of the thermal and circulatory systems during exercise (Herbert, 1983).

Despite the efficiency of the circulating cooling system, the circulating blood cannot keep pace with the body's need to dissipate heat in hot climates and during strenuous exercise. At this point, the second major heat-regulating contribution of water comes into play: *sweat*.

Contrary to popular belief, sweating itself is not what cools the body; it is the *evaporation* of the water in the sweat. In fact, above environmental temperatures of 63° Fahrenheit (17° centigrade), vaporization of sweat is the principal avenue for heat loss during exercise (Mitchell, 1977). This is because it takes energy for water to be changed from its liquid form to water vapor, its gas form. If you fill a pan with water and place it in a room, the water evaporates slowly. If you set the pan on the stove and add heat energy, the water molecules speed up their movements and escape more quickly, hastening evaporation. Heat

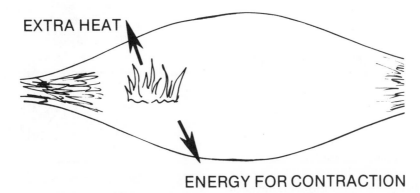

EXTRA HEAT

ENERGY FOR CONTRACTION

Figure 9.4. As the body's cells, including the muscle cells, burn fuel to release energy for life maintenance as well as movement, a great deal of excess heat energy is given off.

from the body does precisely the same thing to the water molecules in the sweat. The body's heat energy supplies the necessary energy to speed up evaporation, and in doing so, heat is lost from the body as water molecules escape to become water vapor.

Water as a Medium for Chemical Reactions

Even though the excess heat energy produced by the chemical reactions taking place in the cells sometimes poses a cooling problem for the body, life would be impossible if those chemical reactions ceased. These reactions are necessary to release the needed energy for life functions, and water is the medium in which these reactions take place. In fact, the higher the reaction rate or metabolic rate within a cell, the greater that cell's water content. This is part of the reason why muscle or lean tissue has a higher water content than does fat tissue; more water is required to carry out the chemical reactions involved in the vigorous functions of the muscle.

The necessary water cannot be available to the muscles or to other cells if athletes lose weight by losing water. Not only do dehydrating practices take water from the blood plasma and other extracellular spaces, they also draw water from the cells themselves. With a diminished water volume, these cells have a diminished capacity to produce energy.

Thus, water is vital to efficient body function, especially for athletes who participate in daily practice sessions that demand lots of energy. Even though a large percent of their body weight is made up of water, these athletes can ill afford to jeopardize their body hydration levels.

DANGERS OF DEHYDRATION

Each of the functions of water we have mentioned is critical, not only to wrestlers who wish to give their "all" on the mat, but also to ice skaters trying to concentrate on mastering an intricate routine, gymnasts who train long hours, and football players who need the stamina to perform in hot, humid weather. For the heart, lungs, and entire circulatory system of these athletes to function optimally, their

blood volume, which is 42% to 50% water, must be adequate. Dehydration refers to the loss of body water from the various body fluid compartments, including the plasma, the water bathing the cells, and the water inside the cells. The reduction of plasma, for example, reduces blood volume. This means that the heart must pump much faster than usual to compensate for the reduced volume of blood, for the blood is faced with the relentless tasks of transporting oxygen and fuel to the engine-like muscle cells as well as removing wastes and by-products. If the muscle cells do not receive enough oxygen and fuel, they will not be able to produce the energy athletes need.

Decreased Cardiovascular Efficiency

Scientists investigated the effects of reduced availability of oxygen during dehydration by first dehydrating athletes and then having them perform various types of hard physical exercise (see Figure 9.5). During these workouts, which included such tasks as running on a treadmill, a special mouthpiece was used to collect air and determine oxygen consumption—that is, how much oxygen was used. After the athlete recovered and rehydrated, the experiment was repeated. Again, the maximum amount of work and the maximum oxygen consumption

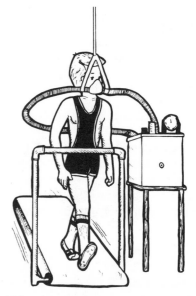

Figure 9.5. Treadmills and other special testing equipment have been used to determine how dehydration influences the muscle's ability to use oxygen to burn fuel.

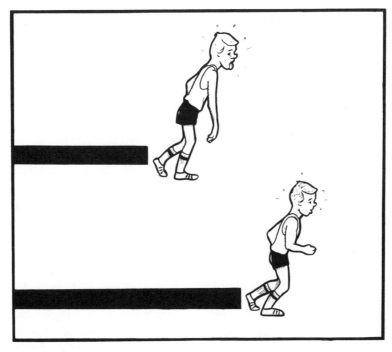

Figure 9.6. Athletes who begin exercise in a dehydrated state (as has the athlete on the top) are unable to work as long as athletes who begin with normal hydration (like the athlete on the bottom).

was recorded. The results led scientists to conclude that although dehydration probably does not reduce the body's capacity to consume a maximal amount of oxygen (Bock, Fox, & Bowers, 1967), it does reduce the amount of time an athlete can work hard before being exhausted (Astrand & Saltin, 1964). This relationship is illustrated in Figure 9.6. These same studies also indicated that the heart of a dehydrated athlete working below his or her maximum must do more work than it would have to do under normal hydration conditions.

Decreased Heat-Regulating Ability

In addition to carrying oxygen, the blood's role in heat removal is particularly important. If this heat is allowed to build, the resultant tissue and enzyme destruction can be lethal. It is vital that the body fluid volumes are not diminished by dehydration.

Decreased Cell Efficiency

As extracellular water is lost during dehydration, the body attempts to balance the water concentration inside and outside the cells, and water is actually drawn from the cells. The cells, including muscle cells, have less water available to support their energy-producing chemical reactions. These chemical reactions are necessary to supply the energy for performing well in sports.

Kidney Damage

Still another harmful effect of decreasing the body's fluid volume is the impact on kidney function. Normally, the kidneys may filter as many as 180 liters of plasma a day (a liter is slightly more than a quart). Most of the filtered plasma goes back into the blood, because the kidney produces only 1 to 1.5 liters of urine daily. This filtration of large quantities of plasma is not a wasted effort, however. In the filtering process, the kidney removes liquid wastes and regulates electrolyte levels (see chapter 10). In fact, the filtration of a certain quantity of plasma is essential if the kidney itself is to remain healthy.

Medical authorities have advised that an individual's daily urine production should not be allowed to fall below 1,200 milliliters. Although it may be impractical to have your athletes measure urine production, they can note the color and odor of their urine. If it is as dilute as it should be, it will be clear, color-less, and relatively odorless. If the athlete is de-hydrated, the kidney will conserve water by producing concentrated, strong-smelling, dark yellow urine. If an athlete is taking water-soluble vitamin supplements, the urine will be yellow; but the volume of urine produced will not decrease. As a result, there will be no strong ammonia smell.

Low urine production is quite likely for the athlete employing rapid weight loss tactics, because fluid restriction and dehydration prac-tices decrease the flow of blood through the kidney (called renal flow). This results in a de-creased volume of fluid filtered by the kidney. Not only may rapid weight loss techniques detract from the athlete's performance, the use of these techniques may be detrimental for a vital organ: the kidney.

Perhaps you are thinking, "But I've seen athletes perform well after dehydrating." Just as there are some athletes who can run faster than others, there are a few athletes whose bodies tolerate dehydrating procedures. These athletes have such talent that they can win in spite of the dehydration, not because they are lighter in weight. Winning despite the de-hydration is possible because the energy-producing machinery does not grind to a halt when the athlete is dehydrated. Therefore, talented athletes can still win, even though the energy-producing system is below par. Unfor-tunately, as long as a few competitors who uti-lize dehydration to "make weight" win their matches, the myths about rapid water weight loss are perpetuated. Knowledgeable coaches must dispel these myths by following the guidelines presented later in this chapter. If coaches of weight-restricted sports (e.g., wres-tling) do this, many youngsters who quit the sport because they can't tolerate using de-hydration as a way of making weight may participate longer.

DEHYDRATING TECHNIQUES

Up to this point, we have talked about the ef-fects of dehydration in a rather general way. An examination of specific dehydrating tech-niques reveals still more reasons why you need to implement steps to prevent your ath-letes from dehydrating themselves.

As has been noted previously, the body's water content is divided into a number of different compartments. The water volume varies from compartment to compartment, and water losses from the various compart-ments can be disproportionate. For example, the dehydration stemming from the use of a diuretic will cause a disproportionate decrease in the plasma water—approximately twice the percentage of body weight lost (Claremont, Costill, Fink, & Van Handel, 1976).

Other research shows that both exercise and thermal dehydration techniques result in very similar fractional reductions in plasma volume that are about twice the percent reduction in body weight. As the water loss exceeds 2% of the body weight the decrease in endurance performance becomes more profound, but muscular strength does not appear to be ham-pered (Herbert, 1983). However, when water loss exceeds 5% of body weight, the ability to sustain near-maximal exercise is diminished (Astrand & Saltin, 1964).

In the past, athletes have employed a variety of tactics for rapidly losing body water. These procedures include

- sweating,
- induced vomiting,
- use of water pills (diuretics),
- use of laxatives (cathartics), and
- expectorating.

For the most part, these tactics reflect exag-gerations of the normal avenues for water loss. Normal daily water losses are usually offset by water consumed through eating and drinking (see Figure 9.7). Even under circumstances of only moderate temperature and light physical activity, enough water is lost that the body's entire water mass must be replaced every 11 to 13 days. Vigorous exercise, high tempera-tures, and high relative humidity result in an even higher turnover rate. By exaggerating the avenues for water loss and restricting their water replacement schedules, athletes have used dehydration as a means of "making weight"—either for specific competition as in wrestling and crew, or just as a means of maintaining their body weight.

We have already described the general dangers of dehydration. Now let's look at the various dehydrating tactics and their specific effects on the body.

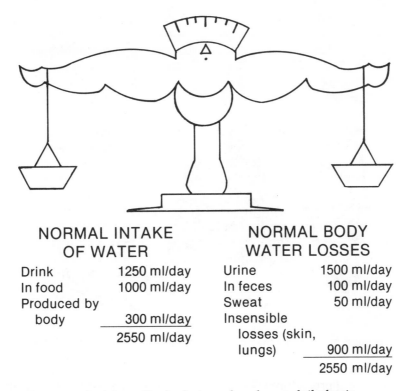

NORMAL INTAKE OF WATER		NORMAL BODY WATER LOSSES	
Drink	1250 ml/day	Urine	1500 ml/day
In food	1000 ml/day	In feces	100 ml/day
Produced by		Sweat	50 ml/day
body	300 ml/day	Insensible	
	2550 ml/day	losses (skin,	
		lungs)	900 ml/day
			2550 ml/day

Figure 9.7. Normally, water lost from the body is replaced on a daily basis.

Sweating

Sweat, the fluid secreted by the sweat glands, contains extracellular water along with small quantities of "salts" (electrolytes). Because the evaporation of sweat provides a means of losing body heat, the onset of sweating is controlled by a thermostat in a part of the brain called the hypothalamus. The thermostat detects when body temperature rises above a specified level and causes sweating to begin and continue until body temperature is reduced or the body's water content is too low to support further sweating. The athlete can reduce body weight significantly by stimulating the sweating mechanism.

This, of course, can be accomplished by engaging in physical activity, being in a hot room or a "sweat box" environment (see Figure 9.8), or a combination of both. Being in a hot room (thermal stress) may further exaggerate water loss from physical activity because it slows heat loss due to the nonsweating avenues, resulting in still more sweating.

Increasing the relative humidity of an environment can impair evaporation. Therefore, standing or exercising in a steam room elevates body temperature and stimulates sweating. The sweat, however, cannot evaporate, allowing little or no cooling effect, so the profuse sweating continues.

When an individual engages in physical activity to induce sweating, some of the energy for the activity is released from the fuel foods, and excess energy builds up as heat in the body, raising the body temperature. When the body temperature reaches a certain level, the hypothalamus initiates sweating. If the sweat evaporates, the skin is cooled and body heat can escape, preventing the body temperature from going too high. The more exercise done, the larger the volume of sweat lost.

Exaggeration of water loss through exercise is accomplished by preventing the evaporation of sweat and the escape of body heat. This procedure is really a combination of thermal stress and exercise stress. By wearing excessive layers of clothing or by increasing the room temperature, the individual uses thermal stress to further stimulate the exercise-induced sweating. Furthermore, wearing excessive clothing can impair the evaporation of

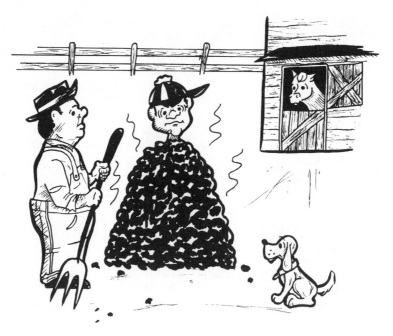

Figure 9.8.   Athletes have been very creative in constructing "sweat boxes" for weight loss.

sweat from the skin. This is particularly true when a person wears rubberized clothing during exercise.

Significant quantities of water can be lost in this fashion, about 2 to 3 liters per hour up to a maximum of 12 liters. In fact, on hot, humid days, up to 20 pounds of water loss have been recorded by some large athletes. Of course, losses of this magnitude seriously jeopardize health; all too frequently, they can result in death from heat stroke. But even less drastic levels of dehydration have been shown to hinder performance. Nonetheless, sweat-induced dehydration is a common practice in certain sports.

Thermal stress can also be dangerous in another way. In response to the heat, blood vessels all over the body's surface dilate, or open up. This allows blood to pass through vessels that are close to the surface, making it easier for the "heat load" to move from the warm blood to a relatively cooler environment. This dilation explains why skin becomes red as the body temperature rises. The red coloration indicates that the blood is merely flowing closer to the surface. If the athlete is submerged in hot water or sitting in a sauna, blood vessels all over the body dilate. It takes a lot of blood to fill all these vessels. Consequently, the amount of blood flowing to the brain is reduced. The result is drowsiness or even unconsciousness. For this reason,

trainers must never leave athletes unattended in hot, whole-body whirlpools; an athlete could easily nod off to sleep, slip under the water, and drown. All too frequently, an athlete who is trying to lose water weight is alone in the steam room, shower, or bathtub. There have been tragic reports of fatalities when athletes passed out and drowned, or passed out and died from head injuries under these conditions. The threat of danger from both the direct and indirect use of thermal stress is very real indeed.

Vomiting

The food we eat goes from the mouth into the stomach rather quickly, but some time passes before the food is digested and its various nutrients are absorbed through the intestinal wall. Some athletes (and their parents) take advantage of this time delay between eating and absorption (see Figure 9.9). This technique allows individuals to experience all the pleasurable sensations associated with eating, but before the food can be moved out of the stomach, a finger or other noxious object is used to induce vomiting. All of the calorie-containing food is ejected from the stomach. In reality, much more than just food is ejected. Large quantities of water and chloride, in the form of hydrochloric acid, and other fluids are excreted

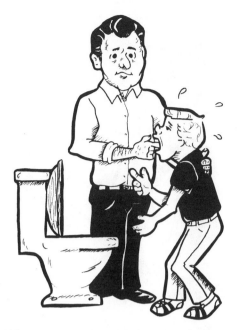

Figure 9.9. Some reports claim that parents take their youngsters' weight control into their own hands.

by the glands in the walls of the stomach to aid in the digestive process. Usually these fluids and many other substances are absorbed in the large and small intestines and therefore not lost from the body. Vomiting, however, results in the loss of large quantities of water and electrolytes as well as food. True, these losses do reduce the body's weight, but they do so at the expense of body water.

In addition to dehydrating the athlete, forced vomiting also causes serious destruction of the body's electrolyte balance (see chapter 10). The hydrochloric acid from the stomach can also damage the athlete's esophagus, mouth, lips, and teeth. The loss of acid also disturbs the body's acid-base balance, adding yet another obstacle to the efficiency of the muscle's energy-producing chemical reactions. For some athletes, forced vomiting may become habitual and lead to an eating disorder called *bulimia*. More information about bulimia and other eating disorders observed in athletes is presented in chapter 12.

Water Pills

The kidney continually filters plasma from the blood, removing waste products and then returning most of the plasma to the blood. The

wastes and plasma water that remain in the kidney are then excreted from the body as urine. The actual volume of urine excreted is under the control of hormones that regulate the reabsorption of filtered plasma. Thus, by influencing reabsorption, urine production may be regulated. The so-called water pill is really a diuretic, a substance that prevents much of the filtered plasma water from being returned to the blood. Several pounds of weight can be lost by taking water pills, but only at the expense of the body's critical water supply (see Figure 9.10).

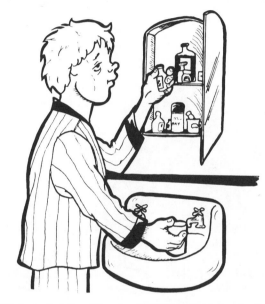

Figure 9.10. The family medicine chest often proves a ready source of water pills.

An individual can also achieve diuretic effects by consuming beverages that contain caffeine, such as coffee, tea, certain cola drinks, and cocoa, instead of actually taking water pills. Emotional stress and nervousness also tend to have diuretic effects and could further compound dehydration and detract from an athlete's performance potential.

Laxatives

As discussed previously, a considerable amount of fluid is secreted by glands in the walls of the stomach, and still more fluids are secreted into the intestine. Normally, the water in these fluids is not lost to the body because 99% of it is reabsorbed in the intestines.

Only 3% to 5% of the daily water loss occurs through the feces. This picture changes dramatically if laxatives or cathartics are taken. These products stimulate the walls of the large intestine to eject wastes before the water can be absorbed. Substantial quantities of body water can be lost in this manner. In addition, not only are the body's water compartments depleted, but substantial potassium and other electrolyte losses occur as well.

Athletes who suffer a bout of diarrhea are left feeling weak and washed-out. Athletes cannot afford to lose these fluids and electrolytes—either voluntarily by taking laxatives or involuntarily through a case of diarrhea (see Figure 9.11)!

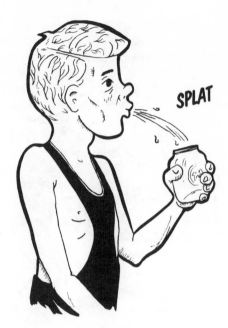

Figure 9.12.   Expectoration is just another way athletes rid themselves of necessary body water.

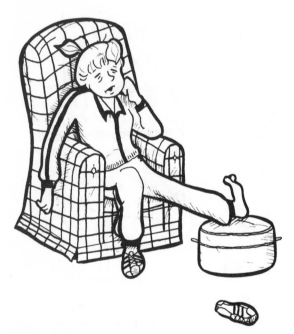

Figure 9.11.   Because laxatives drain athletes' body water and electrolytes, they leave athletes feeling weak and washed out.

Expectoration

The sight of a wrestler spitting into a cup is not uncommon, as this technique is used as a last effort to cut weight (see Figure 9.12). Saliva, or spit, is manufactured by the salivary glands. Water is its primary constituent; thus, repeated spitting or expectoration represents another drain on the body's critical water supply.

PREVENTING DEHYDRATION

Given the possible health and performance hazards associated with dehydration, coaches should take steps to ensure that their athletes do not use any of the above voluntary dehydrating techniques. These same steps also help ensure that involuntary or accidental dehydration does not occur.

Educate Your Athletes

The first step requires that you discuss the detrimental effects of dehydration with your athletes. A little knowledge often goes a long way.

Monitor Body Weight

Because water is quite heavy (a pint weighs about 1 pound), rapid fluctuations in body weight indicate that dehydration is taking place. If you get your athletes in the habit of checking their body weight before and after practices, they will be able to see how much water they have lost, because most of the weight loss will be water weight. Charts for recording pre- and postworkout weights can be obtained free of charge from Cramer Products (P.O. Box 1001, Gardner, KS 66030) and Stokely-VanCamp, Inc. (P.O. Box 1113, Indianapolis, IN 46206). Athletes who lose more than 2% of their body weight from day to day are in jeopardy of involuntary dehydration. Athletes who routinely experience large fluctuations in body weight (6% or more of their body weight) are likely to be using one or more of the dehydrating techniques. These athletes should not be allowed to practice or compete until they can demonstrate more stable daily body weight patterns. In some instances large swings in body weight also indicate certain eating disorders, and these athletes may require professional help. Guidelines for identifying such potential problems are presented in chapter 12.

Encourage Fluid Consumption Before Practice

The consumption of quantities of water before exercise is known as hyperhydrating. The theory is that this procedure temporarily increases the volume of water in the body. Research suggests that this is particularly effective in hot environments and situations where fluid replacement during the activity is difficult (Greenleaf & Castle, 1971). There is, however, a limit to how much water may be consumed without having a diuretic effect. Apparently most athletes may consume 0.5 to 1.0 liters of fluid 20 to 30 minutes or so prior to activity (Williams, 1985). Although such hyperhydrating tactics have been shown to reduce heat stress and improve cardiovascular efficiency, the research relative to beverage consumption shows that optimal hydration is best achieved if fluids are replaced during the exercise.

Have Fluids Available During Practice

Telling your athletes that they need to replace lost fluids is important, but as a coach you also need to make provisions for athletes to replace fluids during the actual practice and training sessions. The following information should help you choose what fluids to use and make decisions about other concerns as well.

Fluids chilled to about 40 to 50 degrees Fahrenheit seem to be absorbed faster (Williams, 1985). The quantity of fluid should be about 6 or 7 ounces at 15- to 20-minute intervals. Athletes will tolerate this drinking best if it is done during practice and training as well as during competitions (Fink, 1982). If the environmental temperature is high and fluid replacement rather than energy replacement is the major goal, the fluid should not be too concentrated. In other words, fluids that have some sugar and electrolytes in them seem to be desirable, but the athlete who puts half a cup of honey in a squirt bottle full of tea is preparing too concentrated a solution. According to the research, beverages that are high in glucose and electrolytes slow gastric (or stomach) emptying, and therefore less-concentrated solutions are preferred. For many years it was thought, as proposed by Coyle, Costill, Fink, & Hoopes (1978), that a 2.5% glucose solution was optimal for rapid absorption. More recently, however, it has been demonstrated that slightly more concentrated drinks (up to 10% glucose) may be appropriate (Lamb & Brodowicz, 1986).

The concentrations of potassium and other electrolytes such as chloride and sodium are also a consideration. Again, if the concentration of these substances is too high, gastric emptying is impaired. Table 9.1 suggests dilution formulas to achieve the appropriate concentration of glucose in various substances (Hackman, 1985).

With some recently developed glucose-polymer solutions (e.g., Excel from Ross Laboratory and Max from the Coca-Cola Company), the rate of gastric emptying is not much different than with water (Wheeler & Banwell, 1986). These beverages seem to be well suited for both fluid and fuel replacement (see chapter 14) and do not need to be diluted.

Because of all the technology that has gone into the development, production, and marketing of the various sports drinks available to today's athletes, these beverages can be quite costly. Cold water, however, is not very expensive at all. Water is readily absorbed, and you don't have to worry about picking a flavor that everyone will like. Even though it doesn't have a fancy name, water is an excellent choice for a fluid replacement drink.

Table 9.1
Dilution Suggestions for Rapid Absorption[1]

Beverages and sugars	Amount	Sugar (grams)	Water to add to achieve a 2.5% sugar solution	Water to add to achieve a 10% sugar solution
Coca-Cola[2]	8 oz	25	25 oz	0.25 oz
Pepsi[2]	8 oz	26	26 oz	0.50 oz
7-Up[2]	8 oz	24	24 oz	0.00 oz
Ginger ale[2]	8 oz	19	18 oz	0.00 oz
Lemonade	8 oz	23	24 oz	0.00 oz
Orange juice (natural)	8 oz	26	26 oz	0.50 oz
Apple juice (natural)	8 oz	29	31 oz	1.75 oz
Table sugar	1 T	12	21 oz	6.0 oz
Fructose	1 T	12	21 oz	6.0 oz
Glucose	1 T	12	21 oz	6.0 oz
Honey	1 T	18	21 oz	6.0 oz

[1]Gatorade and ERG are 5% solutions as sold. They can be diluted to 2.5% solutions by adding 8 ounces of water for each 8 ounces of the product.

[2]Be sure to defizz carbonated beverages.

Require Postexercise Fluid Replacement

Even with the best of fluid replacement schedules, particularly if the exercise is intense (above 70% of maximum), the quantity of body water lost still exceeds the amount replaced. Consequently, postexercise fluid replacement is a must. This replacement should be systematic rather than governed by thirst, because thirst alone takes several days to bring about full restoration (Bar-or, Dotan, Inbar, Rotshtein, & Zonder, 1980). Because we know that a pint of water weighs about a pound, you can use body weight to monitor fluid replacement. This may be done by recording athletes' pre- and postexercise weights. By calculating 2% of the pre-exercise weight, some guidelines for postexercise fluid replacement may be established. (Sources for obtaining charts to record pre- and postexercise weights were cited previously in this chapter.) For example, Marvin weighs 110 pounds (lb) before soccer practice. Two percent of this weight would be

$$110 \text{ lb} \times 0.02 = 2.2 \text{ lb}$$

After practice Marvin weighs 106 lb. He has lost 4 lb of weight during practice, which is more than 2% of his body weight. Most of this is water weight, so before his next practice, Marvin should be back to within 2% of his original weight. At his next prepractice weigh-in, Marvin should weigh no less than 107.8 lb (110 lb − 2.2 lb = 107.8 lb). The difference between his postexercise weight of 106 lb and the value that brings him to within 2% of his original weight (107.8 lb) is 1.8 lb. Marvin should replace this weight by drinking an extra 2 pints of fluid and eating balanced meals, as discussed later in this book. This procedure and the others in this chapter do not guarantee where the body will distribute the water, but they do help the body to establish appropriate hydration levels.

WATER TOXICITY

Although specific water replacement schedules have been shown to help prevent involuntary dehydration (Williams, 1985), forced water consumption should be contingent upon weight loss during exercise. Remember, use a scale to monitor rapid weight loss during a period of physical activity. Then lost water should be replaced at the rate of one pint per pound lost.

If fluid replacement exceeds the volume of water lost due to sweating and other mechanisms, the kidneys may not be able to rid the body of the excess water rapidly enough. The result is that the extracellular sodium is diluted, leading to a condition called *hyponatremia* (low sodium concentration). Its symptoms are disorientation, confusion, restlessness, increased temperature, increased heart rate, and increased blood pressure.

Several cases of such water toxicity have been reported (Frizzell, Lang, Lowance, & Lathan, 1986) in association with endurance events. The American Medical Joggers Association recommends that you check for weight loss, indicative of dehydration, or weight gain, indicative of hyponatremia. Using a weight chart to record pre- and postexercise body weights, as suggested previously in this chapter, should prevent the occurrence of water toxicity.

SUMMARY AND RECOMMENDATIONS

A considerable portion of the body weight of lean, conditioned athletes is water weight, but this does not represent excess weight. Water plays a significant role in the function of the body, and the healthy athlete really does not have any water to spare. This is especially true for young athletes (American Academy of Pediatrics, 1982). Dehydration can have serious consequences whether it is done purposefully by a wrestler trying to make weight or whether it occurs by accident because proper preventive strategies were not followed. To ensure that your athletes are well hydrated, you must take the following steps:

1. Inform your athletes about the consequences of dehydration.
2. Require that your athletes monitor their body weight before and after every exercise session.
3. Encourage athletes to get in the habit of hyperhydrating before exercise.
4. Provide cold fluids for athletes to consume during practice and training sessions.
5. Require that athletes rehydrate back to within 2% of their pre-exercise body weight.

Chapter 10
Electro-Whats?

Along with understanding the vital role of water, you need to understand what electrolytes are and what roles they play in body function. We used the term *electrolyte* in discussing dehydration and fluid replacement strategies in the preceding chapter, but we did not explain what electrolytes are or why they are necessary.

An electrolyte is not a new wonder drug that scientists have just discovered, nor is it a miracle food additive that assures athletic prowess. An electrolyte is a charged molecule. Normally, most molecules are neutral; that is, they have an equal number of positive protons and negative electrons. Table salt, for instance, is chemically represented by the symbol NaCl, with the Na standing for sodium (natrium) and the Cl for chloride. Sodium chloride does not have an electrical charge, but when placed in water, as in Figure 10.1, the sodium and chloride molecules separate, producing two electrolytes: Na$^+$ and Cl$^-$. These charged molecules, and others, have important roles to play in various life functions, so it is absolutely essential that the body maintain appropriate quantities of electrolytes.

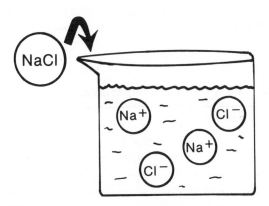

Figure 10.1. When salt (NaCl) is placed in water, it separates into two electrolytes: Na$^+$ and Cl$^-$.

SOURCES OF ELECTROLYTES

Maintaining appropriate quantities of electrolytes is an ongoing process, because the body loses electrolytes through several pathways. One of the most obvious is sweat. You have no doubt noticed sweat's salty taste. Recognition of the loss of Na$^+$, Cl$^-$, and other electrolytes in sweat has prompted some athletes to use salt tablets and electrolyte drinks as replacement strategies. It is also possible to replenish the body's electrolyte supply with a diet that includes fruits, vegetables, grains, and meats. These foods provide the necessary electrolytes (sodium = Na$^+$; potassium [kalium] = K$^+$; chloride = Cl$^-$; calcium = Ca^{2+}; magnesium = Mg^{2+}; hydrogen = H$^+$). Whether electrolyte supplements and electrolyte drinks are necessary for the athlete and whether natural foods can be utilized to maintain electrolyte balances are addressed in the remaining sections of this chapter.

WHERE ARE THE ELECTROLYTES?

Once ingested, electrolytes can be found in a number of locations throughout the fluid compartments of the body. Interestingly, electrolytes do not appear in equal concentrations in the different compartments. Some electrolytes are located predominantly in the extracellular fluids, and others are primarily in the intracellular fluids. Sodium and potassium are the two electrolytes found in the highest concentrations in the body fluids, but even these two are not located in the same fluid spaces. Higher concentrations of sodium (Na$^+$) are found in the extracellular fluids, whereas potassium (K$^+$) can be found in larger quantities inside the cells. This difference in the relative

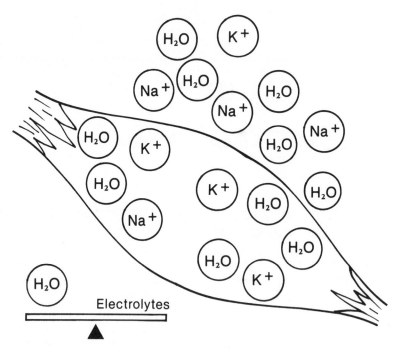

Figure 10.2. The total concentration of electrolytes on either side of the cell's membrane must be "balanced" for life functions to continue.

concentrations of various electrolytes is funda-mental to life, because without such a balance between the inside and outside of cells, nerves would be unable to send impulses, skeletal muscles would be unable to contract, and even the heart would stop pumping. This balance of water and electrolytes is portrayed in Figure 10.2. Table 10.1 shows the precise concentrations of three of the major electrolytes.

For life functions to proceed optimally, it is critical that the relatively large concentration of potassium inside the cells be offset or balanced by the sodium concentration outside. If this balance is disturbed, body functions will deteriorate accordingly—a fate that athletes can ill afford if they wish to perform

to peak capacity (Van Itallie, Sinisterra, & Stare, 1960).

EFFECTS OF EXERCISE ON ELECTROLYTE DISTRIBUTION

During exercise or physical work, a series of dynamic changes normally occurs in the distribution of the body's water. When the activity begins, water is immediately transferred from the extracellular fluid into the muscle cells (Wilkerson, Horvath, Gutin, Molnar, & Diaz, 1982) (see Figure 10.3). This transfer of water

Table 10.1
Distribution of Various Electrolytes in the Body's Fluid Compartments

Electrolyte	Extracellular compartment (millimoles/L of H_2O)	Intracellular compartment (millimoles/L of H_2O)
NA^+	150	15
Cl^-	125	10
K^+	5	150

AT REST

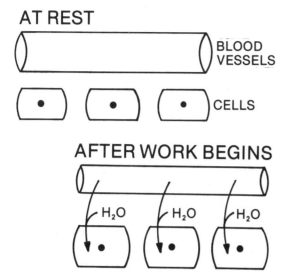

Figure 10.3. During exercise, a characteristic shift in the body's water distribution occurs.

facilitates the energy-producing chemical reactions, discussed in chapter 5, that take place in the muscle cells. The extracellular fluid that moves into the muscles is rapidly replaced by water from the blood plasma. Under normal conditions, the accompanying small decrease in blood volume is tolerable because it plays a role in increasing the water in the cell, thus increasing the energy-producing capabilities of the muscle cells.

Increased Sodium Outside of Cells

The shifting of body water into cells depends on a delicate balance of the electrolytes in the various compartments. This is because electrolytes are not usually free to move across membranes, and therefore water is drawn across membranes to equalize concentrations. The greater the difference in the concentration of electrolytes on either side of a membrane, the greater the pressure drawing the water across the membrane to dilute the concentration of electrolytes (osmotic pressure). For example, if an excessive amount of table salt (NaCl) were consumed, as shown in the upper half of Figure 10.4, the concentration of Na^+ in the extracellular spaces would temporarily increase—until the regulatory mechanisms had time to remove the excess Na^+. Because very little Na^+ is allowed to cross the cell membranes, the concentration of sodium in the intracellular spaces would not be altered. Thus,

as a result of consuming excess salt, the high concentration of sodium in the extracellular spaces is temporarily larger than normal. The high concentration of sodium in the extracellular spaces draws H_2O from the intracellular compartment to dilute the excessive number of Na^+ ions in the extracellular space and maintain the proper concentration balance, as shown in the bottom of Figure 10.4.

Decreased Cellular Water

Such a water shift is completed at the expense of the cell's water, which, as you remember, is critical for the chemical reactions that produce energy. Theoretically, then, this elevation of the sodium concentration in the extracellular fluid impairs physical performance because it prevents the shift of water into muscle cells. The word theoretical is used because current research information does not clearly indicate how such electrolyte disturbances influence the biochemical processes in the exercising muscle (Herbert, 1983).

Water Losses With Sweating

The athlete who loses a great deal of water due to sweating (5 to 8 pounds) creates a similar situation. Sweating not only results in the loss of body water; it also disturbs the body's electrolyte balance because sweat is *hypotonic*, which means that it is primarily water, not salt. When the salt concentration in sweat is compared to the concentration of salt in the extracellular fluid, the sweat is very dilute (thus the term hypotonic). The sweat of an athlete who is accustomed (or acclimatized) to working in the heat is even more hypotonic (diluted).

Unfortunately, many coaches believe that sweat contains lots of salt. This is not true. In fact, as athletes sweat, they lose relatively more water than electrolytes, and the fluid that is left in the extracellular spaces becomes more and more concentrated with electrolytes. Again, to reduce this electrolyte concentration, water is drawn out of the cells, as shown in Figure 10.5, to dilute the extracellular fluid. As a result, during exercise the cells may well be deprived of necessary water (L. Rose, Carroll, Lowe, Peterson, & Cooper, 1970).

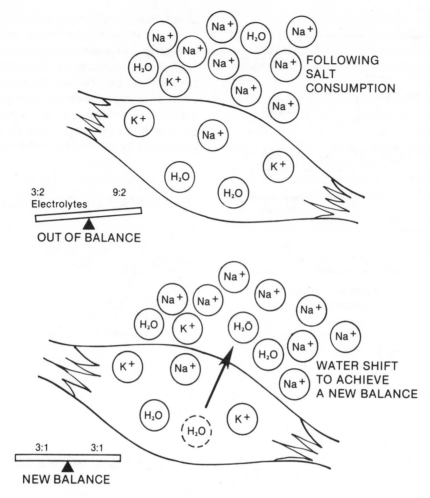

Figure 10.4. Consumption of excessive salt (NaCl) results in an increased concentration of sodium (Na^+) in the extracellular space, which draws water out of the cells to regain a concentration balance.

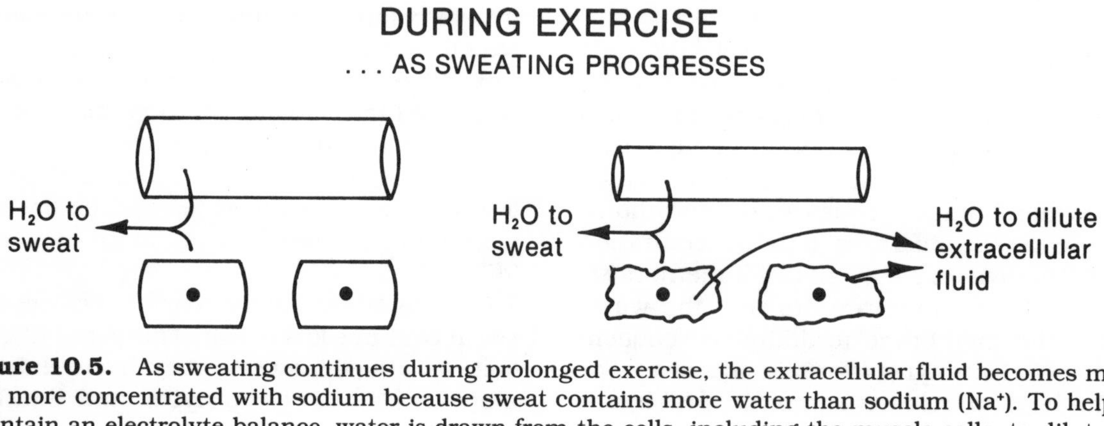

DURING EXERCISE
. . . AS SWEATING PROGRESSES

H_2O to sweat

H_2O to sweat

H_2O to dilute extracellular fluid

Figure 10.5. As sweating continues during prolonged exercise, the extracellular fluid becomes more and more concentrated with sodium because sweat contains more water than sodium (Na^+). To help maintain an electrolyte balance, water is drawn from the cells, including the muscle cells, to dilute the extracellular fluid.

SODIUM REPLACEMENT

It should now be obvious how consuming salt tablets often makes the decreased cellular water condition even worse, particularly if they are taken while exercising (Cade, 1971). Instead of helping the balance, further increased concentration of Na^+ in the extracellular fluid resulting from the ingestion of salt tablets temporarily disrupts the system by drawing needed water from the muscle cells. Several authorities have also suggested that excessive Na^+ intake may disturb normal potassium balance (Costill, 1972; Williams, 1985).

A person's average daily salt consumption is about 10 to 12 grams, which equals about 4.0 to 4.8 grams of Na^+ per day. It is possible, however, to lose up to 5 to 7 grams of Na^+ (along with 11 to 18 pounds of fluid) under extreme heat and exercise conditions (Verde, Shephard, Corey, & Moore, 1982). Under these extreme conditions, some Na^+ supplementation may be needed, but conditions are rarely this extreme. With daily exercise, particularly in the heat, the body begins to retain more Na^+ than normal (9 grams over 5 days) (Costill, Branam, Fink, & Nelson, 1976). Obviously, then, sodium replacement is necessary only if large amounts of water weight are lost through sweat. There are four potential strategies for replacing excessive Na^+ losses: the use of salt tablets, electrolyte drinks, extra table salt, and foods containing sodium.

Salt Tablets

Although salt tablets have been around for many years, they have been and continue to be misused because some athletes take them even with small weight losses. The tablets are also frequently taken with little or no water, so they result in temporary but substantial increases in extracellular sodium. In addition to potentially impairing physical performance, elevated sodium concentration (*hypernatremia*) can impair heart function (Guyton, 1981). Consequently, the pumping action of the heart stops, causing death. Further, an imbalance in the Na^+: K^+ ratio can also result in death, although a more likely outcome is cramping of skeletal muscles (Costill, Jansson, Gollnick, & Saltin, 1974).

The ingestion of salt tablets can also irritate the walls of the stomach and result in nausea. Using coated, time-release tablets may help with the problem of gastric distress. Even if such time-release tablets are used, coaches who choose to have their athletes use salt

Table 10.2
The Use of Salt Tablets for Sodium Replacement

Losses due to sweating				Replacement need[1]	
Water losses	Salt losses				
Pounds or pints	Grams	Grains	Water to be replaced (pints)	Number of 7-grain salt tablets to be taken per pt H_2O[2]	
				Nonacclimatized	Acclimatized
2	1.5	23	2	0	0
4	3.0	46	4	0	0
6	4.5	69	6	0	0
8	6.0	92	8	2	1
10	7.5	115	10	4	3
12	9.0	138	12	6	5

Note. From *The Physiological Basis of Physical Education and Athletics* by E.L. Fox and D.K. Mathews, copyright © 1976 by Harcourt Brace Jovanovich, Inc., reprinted by permission of the publisher.

[1]Because sweat contains both electrolytes and water, both need to be replaced.

[2]A 7-grain salt tablet contains about ½ grams of salt, or 0.2 grams of Na^+.

tablets should insist that athletes follow the replacement guidelines in Table 10.2 (Fox & Mathews, 1976). Notice that these guidelines say that salt tablets should not be taken until significant fluid losses (8 pounds of sweat weight) have occurred. Also, the guidelines stipulate that each salt tablet must be taken with a pint of water.

Electrolyte Drinks

The use of electrolyte drinks represents another approach to electrolyte replacement. Because the consumption of fluid along with the electrolytes ensures sufficient water intake, these beverages have become very popular and relieve the coach of the burden of watching athletes to make sure they consume water with their salt tablets. Whether these drinks enhance biochemical function during physical activity is difficult to say given the research techniques currently available. According to researchers who have observed athletes' performance parameters while systematically administering various electrolyte drinks, hypotonic (diluted) NaCl drinks are associated with better maintenance of plasma volume and circulatory function during exercise than is water alone (Nose, Mack, Shi, & Nadel, 1988). Conversely, hypertonic (highly concentrated) salt drinks are associated with impairments in heat regulation (Herbert, 1983).

The Salt-Shaker Approach

Because of the potential for abusing salt tablets and because of the cost of providing electrolyte drinks, Williams (1985) and other

Table 10.3
Natural Sources of Sodium and Potassium

Quantity	Source	Sodium (mg)	Potassium (mg)
1	Apple	1.5	180
1 c	Apple juice	2	250
3	Apricots	1	301
1 serving	Asparagus	1	110
1	Banana	1	440
1 slice	Bread (whole wheat)	148	72
½ c	Broccoli (frozen)	14	200
1	Carrot	34	246
2 pieces	Chicken (roasted white meat)	32	206
½ c	Corn (frozen)	1	150
10	Dates	1	518
½ c	Green beans (frozen)	0.5	102
¼ lb	Hamburger	44	203
½ c	Kidney beans	3	315
1	Orange	3	312
1 c	Pineapple juice	3	373
1	Potato (baked)	6	782
3 oz	Round steak	60	272
⅓ c	Raisins	12	328
½ c	Squash (cooked)	1	140
1 c	Spaghetti with meat sauce	1,000	665
1	Tomato	3	222

authorities have suggested that athletes freely salt their food. Though such a strategy will provide adequate NaCl, the athlete may develop a taste for salty food; when training stops, the habit of using extra salt will be difficult to break. For some individuals, excessive salt intake is linked to hypertension, and therefore a lifelong habit of using a lot of salt may be inappropriate for some athletes. Consequently, the use of food for electrolyte replacement is gaining popularity.

The Food Approach

The fourth and final approach to sodium replacement involves having your athletes increase their consumption of fruits and vegetables that naturally contain sodium and other electrolytes. Examples of such fruits and vegetables are presented in Table 10.3. In addition, the judicious consumption of foods that have salt added during processing, such as those listed below can also add sodium to the diet.

Processed Foods That Are High in Salt

Anchovies	Meat tenderizer
Bacon	Mustard
Barbecue sauce	Olives
Beans, butter	Peanut butter
Beans, dried lima	Pickles
Bologna and other luncheon meats	Potato chips and corn chips
Bouillon	Pretzels
Bread and rolls (especially those with salt toppings)	Relishes
	Salt pork
	Salted nuts
Catsup	Salted popcorn
Cheese, American	Salty and smoked fish
Cheese, Swiss	Salty and smoked meat
Cheese, cheddar	Sardines
Chili sauce	Sauerkraut
Chipped and corned beef	Sausage
Cottage cheese	Seasoning (salt, monosodium glutamate, poultry seasoning, etc.)
Crackers	
Diet soda pop	
Dry cereals	Soups (canned)
French fries	Soy sauce
Ham	Tuna and other canned fish
Herring	
Horseradish	Vegetables (canned)
Hot dogs	Worcestershire sauce
Kale	
Kosher meat	

In our opinion, all coaches should adopt the food approach to sodium replacement. The research of Costill, Cote, Miller, Miller, & Wynder (1975) supports this position. They observed that the addition of electrolytes to drinking water was of minimal value, under conditions of moderate dehydration, when the athletes were allowed to eat and drink freely. Dressendorfer et al. (1982) also reported that the endurance runners they observed did not need to consume special electrolyte solutions as long as they consumed well-balanced meals that met their caloric needs.

POTASSIUM IMBALANCE

So far, our discussion of electrolytes has centered on sweating and its potential disruption of the body's sodium balance. Sodium, however, is not the only electrolyte that may become imbalanced, nor is sweating the only means by which the body's electrolyte balances can be disturbed. Human sweat also contains potassium (K^+), along with some other elements. Apparently, potassium losses in sweat are negligible under any but the most extreme conditions (Consolazio, Matoush, Nelson, Harding, & Canaham, 1963). Consequently, sweat-induced potassium depletion is not a primary concern, and a well-balanced diet should adequately restore the potassium that is lost in sweat.

Hyperkalemia

In fact, if K^+ is supplemented too aggressively during exercise, a situation called *hyperkalemia* can arise. During exercise, the concentration of K^+ in the blood rises. This is due partly to the loss of fluid from the plasma and partly to the release of potassium from the muscle cells (Hazeyama & Sparks, 1979). Because of this increase in extracellular potassium during exercise, potassium supplements in addition to normal dietary consumption are discouraged, as they may further increase the exercise-induced increase in extracellular potassium to the point where severe hyperkalemia results. Severe hyperkalemia can be very dangerous, resulting in cardiac arrhythmias (Williams, 1985).

Hypokalemia

While severe hyperkalemia has been reported during both anaerobic and aerobic exercise, there are also reports of *hypokalemia* after exercise. Hypokalemia refers to a low concentration of potassium in the plasma. Although little K^+ is lost in sweat, Knochel (1977) has hypothesized that repeated bouts of intense exercise may result in potassium deficiencies. In addition to the potassium lost in sweat, the body's regulatory mechanism for saving sodium results in the excretion of potassium in urine. Because of this, hypokalemia is especially likely to occur with aggressive sodium supplementation (Costill, 1972).

Potassium Replacement

Much less attention has been focused on potassium replacement than on sodium replacement, but not because K^+ is any less important. Potassium balance is vital to life and important for the optimal functioning of muscles and nerves. Based upon the increased potassium losses noted in exercising athletes, Cade, Spooner, Schlein, Pickering, & Dean (1972) recommend that athletes exercising in the heat need 6 grams of potassium per day. Essentially the same replacement choices that were discussed for Na^+ are also available for potassium.

Potassium Tablets

Although potassium tablets are available, their use poses the risk of hyperkalemia. Therefore, it is suggested that athletes not use potassium tablets (Lane & Cerda, 1979; K. Rose, 1975).

Electrolyte Drinks

Commercial electrolyte drinks contain potassium as well as sodium. Because water is consumed along with the potassium, overdosing is less likely than with tablets. The cost of the drinks is one drawback to this replacement approach, but a more important criticism of using these special drinks to replace electrolytes is that athletes may be less likely to eat a balanced variety of foods.

The Salt-Shaker Approach

Salt substitutes, consisting of potassium chloride (KCl) (made for people on sodium-free diets), are available. Again these products should be used with caution because of the possibility of hyperkalemia (Williams, 1985). A disadvantage to the use of salt substitutes, as well as special drinks, to replace electrolytes is that athletes may not learn the importance of foods as electrolyte sources.

The Food Approach

You can circumvent the drawbacks involved with the three preceding potassium replacement approaches if you have your athletes use food to replace potassium lost during exercise. The replacement requirement of 6 grams per day is at the upper end of the estimated safe and adequate dietary range for potassium suggested by the National Research Council (1980). An individual can easily achieve this goal of 6 grams daily by eating a diet high in fruits, vegetables, and lean meats. For example, an athlete who eats one banana and a small package of raisins as snacks during the day adds nearly a gram of potassium to the diet (one banana = 440 milligrams [mg]; 3 ounces of raisins = 328 mg for a total of 768 mg; remember that 1,000 mg = 1 gram). The potassium contents of some other foods are listed in Table 10.3 (see p. 88).

OTHER ELECTROLYTE IMBALANCES

As stated earlier in this chapter, Na^+ and K^+ are not the only two electrolytes in the body fluids, but they have received the most attention and research. Less is known about replacement strategies for the other electrolytes. We do know, however, that foods are rich sources of electrolytes. That is one of the reasons why so many authorities favor a balanced diet as the preferred method for replacing sodium and potassium. Eating high-quality fruits, vegetables, and other foods on a regular basis ensures that sodium and potassium as well as substantial quantities of the other electrolytes will be ingested. Of course, the other variable is adequate water consumption.

IMBALANCED DIETS AND DEHYDRATING SITUATIONS

Although substantial potassium losses are not likely to occur from exercise-induced sweating and the normal regulatory functions of the kidney, if starvation diets, cathartics, or diuretics are used to effect rapid weight losses, the drain on the body's potassium can be significant. Caloric restriction makes it impossible to use food to replace the lost electrolytes. Under these circumstances, the indiscriminate use of Na^+ and K^+ supplements can be particularly dangerous (Williams, 1985).

Starvation Diets

Stringent dieting can contribute to dehydration and electrolyte imbalances, especially if the athlete is also engaged in training and therefore producing sweat. Because food intake is severely restricted, the loss of electrolytes is not likely to be fully replaced. If the athlete restricts water intake as well, the ensuing dehydration further compromises the body's electrolyte balance. The indiscriminate use of electrolyte supplements under these circumstances is dangerous and can result in heat injuries (Costill, 1972) and other serious consequences for the athlete.

Forced Vomiting

Forced vomiting, which results in the ejection of the chyme (partially digested food) from the stomach, is also associated with substantial losses of water and hydrochloric acid, which contains hydrogen and chloride ions. Some sodium and potassium are also lost in this manner. Additional negative effects of forced vomiting are discussed in chapter 12.

Cathartics

Cathartics (laxatives) stimulate the early elimination of solid waste materials in the large intestine. When solid wastes are eliminated too soon, considerable quantities of potassium and water do not have time to be absorbed and thus are lost from the body. The use of cathartics can bring about dehydration and serious disruption of the body's potassium levels.

The nervous tension that frequently accompanies competition may cause neurogenic diarrhea. This type of diarrhea is the result of excessive stimulation of the parasympathetic nervous system, which greatly excites both the motility of the intestine and the secretion of mucous into the large intestine. These two effects can cause the rapid movement of the waste material through the large intestine, resulting in the loss of large quantities of water and potassium as well as other electrolytes.

The potassium deficiencies resulting from cathartics, neurogenic diarrhea, or any other causes of diarrhea affect the muscles and are characterized by muscular weakness that can result in paralysis. The effects of the potassium deficiency on the smooth muscles that line the walls of the stomach and intestine are diarrhea and intestinal distention. Such a K^+ deficiency may also cause general weakness in the heart and the muscles lining the blood vessels. Obviously, then, severe potassium depletion detracts from physical performance and may even lead to death.

Diuretics

One of the general functions of the electrolytes is to help maintain the body's water balance. Sodium has a particularly important role to play in this regard. If the concentration of sodium falls, the kidney merely excretes water until the proper concentration of sodium and water is reestablished. The kidney excretes water as urine only until the appropriate Na^+ concentration in the extracellular fluid has been reached. Obviously, if the kidney is stimulated to excrete extra Na^+, water is also excreted so that the concentration of Na^+ in the body fluids does not decrease.

Diuretics, or water pills, effectively increase water losses by increasing the volume of urine excreted. In doing so, the diuretic must also stimulate the excretion of sodium, or else the water filtered by the kidney is merely reabsorbed into the extracellular compartment. Because chloride passively follows the sodium ions across the tubules in the kidney, any increase in the excretion of sodium by the kidney results in a corresponding increase in the chloride ions excreted in the urine, resulting in an imbalance of both chloride and sodium.

Diuretics can also disrupt the body's potassium concentration. In fact, individuals who take diuretics as part of their therapy to regulate hypertension (high blood pressure) are also instructed to take medications that contain potassium to avoid potassium deficiency. These people are under proper medical supervision; they are not self-diagnosing their potassium supplementation. It is totally inappropriate and dangerous for athletes to use diuretics or any other dehydrating strategies to lose weight and then try to offset electrolyte losses with supplements.

SUMMARY AND RECOMMENDATIONS

Thermal stress, starvation dieting, forced vomiting, laxatives, and diuretics can all seriously disrupt the body's electrolyte balance and fluid volume. Consequently, they have no place in the weight control practices of athletes young or old. The regulation of body water through such unnatural tactics is not the way to control weight. Furthermore, the indiscriminate use of supplements to counter elec-

trolyte losses incurred by the use of water pills, laxatives, and forced vomiting is dangerous. To ensure that your athletes do not have problems with electrolyte imbalance, you should take the following steps:

1. Maintain pre- and postexercise weight recording charts as discussed in the previous chapter. The use of such charts affords a mechanism for detecting water weight losses, which, if left unchecked, result in electrolyte imbalance as well as hypohydration.

2. Establish specific instructions so that your athletes rehydrate to within 2% of their original pre-exercise weight. If fat loss is a goal, this 2% margin allows athletes to gradually reduce their weight by losing fat, not water.

3. Encourage extra water consumption at the rate of 1 pint per pound of lost weight. If electrolyte drinks are available, a pint or two of these drinks can be substituted for some of the water.

4. Convey the importance of food sources for electrolyte replacement by posting instructions encouraging the consumption of citrus fruits and bananas as snacks and at meals. For example, one high school coach in Wisconsin displays a sign indicating that "A banana a day keeps the cramps away" as a technique for emphasizing the importance of potassium replacement.

PART III
Using Your Knowledge

Chapter 11
How to Lose Fat Weight

As you learned in chapter 1, optimal body weight and physical efficiency go hand in hand. You read about the coach who knew that body composition appraisal and sound nutritional practices would help his athletes enhance their performance potential. To help you toward this goal, body composition appraisal and the prediction of optimal weight were discussed in chapter 2. Then, to provide you with some background information about the basics of good nutrition, chapter 3 discussed the concept of a balanced diet, chapter 4 discussed the importance of carbohydrates and fats, and chapter 5 covered how the cells are able to convert the food that we eat to the energy for physical activity. Chapters 6 through 10 dealt with the important nutritional components of a balanced diet in more detail, giving special attention to how they contribute to body function, particularly in athletes. Now you will learn how to use all of that information to help each of your athletes achieve optimal weight and performance.

CALORIC BALANCE AND BODY COMPOSITION

As a first step, you must determine each athlete's optimal weight by using the caliper technique described in chapter 2. Then you need to understand the relationship between caloric imbalance and body composition.

As long as caloric intake is balanced by caloric expenditure and this balance has existed for some time, body weight remains constant, and the relative amount of fat weight and lean tissue weight stays the same as well. If caloric intake is sharply curtailed and activity level

is unchanged, body weight drops, but much of the weight loss comes from lean tissue weight rather than fat weight. The lean tissue cells are responsible for athletic performance; they are the cells that burn fuels to provide energy for nerves to send impulses and for muscles to contract. Consequently, most athletes cannot afford to lose lean tissue weight.

Losing Excess Weight

Instead, achievement of optimal physical efficiency comes with minimizing excess fat weight. *Fat* is the important word, not just weight. Although crash dieting and dehydrating techniques can have a significant impact on body weight, they have relatively little impact upon the body's fat weight (see Figure 11.1).

Optimal Weight

Optimal body weight, which is associated with optimal performance, can be achieved only by understanding the concept of nutritional balance. An understanding of this balance allows you to manipulate the body's fat weight by regulating the caloric balance and keeping the nutrients in balance as well (see Figure 11.2).

Balancing Calories

Let's first examine the factors that influence caloric balance. These factors include caloric input (the amount of kilocalories consumed)

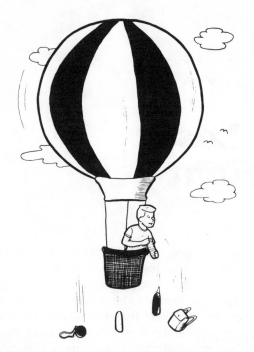

Figure 11.1. When balloonists have to lighten the load, not all weight is considered excess weight. They cannot afford to sacrifice their burners or their fuel. Similarly, athletes should not think of water as excess weight; rather, they should be concerned with minimizing excess fat weight.

and caloric expenditure (the level of physical activity). If these two factors are out of balance, either the fat stores or the lean weight will be affected. Because the proportion of fat and lean weight is so important for optimal physical performance, coaches need to know how caloric imbalances influence an athlete's fat weight and lean weight.

Increasing Stored Fat

If you consume more kilocalories than your body requires, the scale is "tipped" (see Figure 11.3). The extra kilocalories are stored as fat in the adipose or fat cells, causing body composition to change. This increase in stored fat means that the percent of body fat goes up. If the level of physical activity is also reduced, the muscles become smaller and do not weigh as much as before. Therefore, a decrease in level of activity coupled with increased caloric intake can result in a much faster rise in percent fat than occurs if just too many kilocalories are consumed. Furthermore, body weight is affected differently by these two sets of circumstances.

If you increase your caloric consumption and maintain the same level of physical activity, your body weight goes up as you gain fat pounds. But if caloric consumption increases and physical activity decreases, total body weight may not increase a great deal at first, because fat gains are offset by losses of lean or muscle tissue. In other words, the increases in body weight due to stored fat are partially offset by the losses in lean or muscle tissue resulting from the decrease in physical activity. So while there is definitely an imbalance between caloric consumption and physical activity, body weight does not actually tell you how damaging this imbalance is, be-

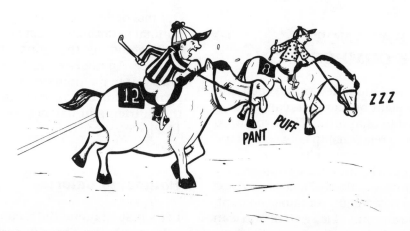

Figure 11.2. Optimal performance efficiency is the result of optimal fat control. A fat horse is unlikely to cross the finish line first, but even so, seldom are scrawny, dehydrated horses found in the winner's circle.

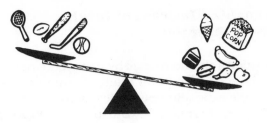

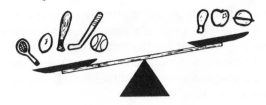

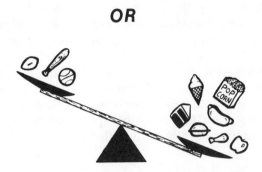

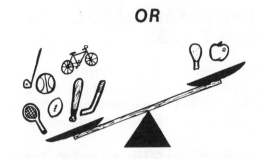

High physical activity with increased consumption

OR

Decreased physical activity and increased consumption

Same physical activity with decreased consumption

OR

Increased physical activity and decreased consumption

Figure 11.3. Body fat is increased by increasing caloric consumption. An even faster increase in body fat occurs if increased caloric consumption is accompanied by decreased activity.

Figure 11.4. Fat loss occurs if caloric consumption is lower than caloric expenditure, and an even more rapid fat loss occurs if caloric restriction is accompanied by increased caloric expenditure.

cause the weight shown on the scale does not measure body composition.

Decreasing Stored Fat

Decreasing caloric intake may tip the balance in the opposite direction (see Figure 11.4). Again, the effect of this procedure on body fat can be misleading if the level of physical activity as well as the amount of decrease in caloric consumption are not taken into account. For example, if the kilocalories consumed, especially carbohydrates, decrease markedly, and the physical activity level is not very high, the body weight drops, but the loss represents lean tissue as well as fat. Under these circumstances, the decrease in the number of kilocalories eaten is not sufficient to cover the caloric costs of the athlete's day-to-day activities. A low carbohydrate intake in particular may result in lower blood sugar levels. The body, however, has a backup mechanism, a safety device for just such occasions. The low number of carbohydrate kilocalories being consumed causes the blood sugar level to drop, and this triggers the release of several hormones. These hormones are very impor-

tant; they allow the muscles to burn their stored glycogen and fat (see chapter 4).

They also allow the liver to release its stored glucose to supply the nerves and brain with fuel. In addition, some of these hormones (the glucocorticoids) break down the proteins in the muscle and other lean tissues. The amino acids from these tissue proteins are then taken into the blood to the liver, where the liver converts them into glucose. Thus, even after the liver's initial glycogen (stored glucose) levels are depleted, the liver can continue to supply glucose to the blood so that the cells of the nervous system have adequate fuel. This process of breaking down protein is so effective that the liver can actually make more glucose than the nerve tissue can use. The "extra" glucose is converted to fat and stored.

Dieting and Fat Loss

Surprising as it may seem, dieting, especially crash dieting, can actually *increase* the body's fat content. Although body weight decreases with this kind of diet, the percent fat increases. Such a situation certainly does not enhance an athlete's physical efficiency, and therefore, the resultant weight should not be considered optimal. Furthermore, a food's kilocalorie content is the only thing that matters in crash diets; therefore, the athlete's restriction of caloric consumption causes nutrient intake to suffer. Remember, for optimal performance, food needs to provide nutrients as well as kilocalories for energy.

NUTRITIONAL GUIDELINES FOR FAT LOSS

We present the following nutritional guidelines for fat loss to help ensure that both of these functions of food are achieved while the body's fat stores are being manipulated.

Nutritional Guidelines for Fat Loss

Lose fat, not muscle

Combine decreased intake with exercise

Reduce body fat gradually

Vary requirements for different individuals

Eat a balanced diet

Drink water

Lose Fat, Not Muscle

Weight loss should come from the fat stores in the body. Losing only fat weight helps ensure physical efficiency. The amount of fat weight that the athlete needs to lose must be approximated by evaluating body fat content as described in chapter 2. By following those procedures you can tell athletes about how many pounds of fat they should lose. For example, in chapter 2 we used the caliper technique to find that Eric, a high school middle-distance runner, had a current percent fat of 14%. Because this percentage is higher than the optimal range of 7% to 12%, it follows that some fat loss would help Eric's performance potential. By doing the calculations presented in the recording form included in chapter 2, we determined that Eric needed to lose abut 3 pounds of fat to reduce his percent fat to 12%. Of course this estimation assumes that Eric's lean weight stays the same.

Combine Decreased Intake With Exercise

Athletes should reduce by using both reduced caloric consumption (dieting) and increased caloric expenditure (physical activity) (Povlou, Steffee, Lerman, & Burrows, 1985). This guideline helps to ensure that the weight loss comes from the body's fat stores, *not* from the lean tissue.

Long-duration, low-intensity activity is probably best for maximizing fat losses (Girandola, 1976). This type of training is best done in the off-season for athletes involved in anaerobic sports, because if too much low-intensity, long-duration exercise is done during the regular season, the anaerobic sport athlete's performance potential will suffer.

Reduce Body Fat Gradually

The caloric balance should be adjusted so that fat losses never exceed 4 pounds per week. A weekly fat loss of 1 to 2 pounds is actually more desirable unless the athlete is very large or consumes more than 5,000 kilocalories each day. The caloric restriction of 2,000 kilocalories per day that is necessary to effect a 4-pound-per-week fat loss in a smaller athlete will stimulate the body's protective mechanism, which causes the breakdown of lean tissue proteins. If the athlete is younger than 15 or 16 years of age, even 2 pounds per week may be excessive (Mann, 1977). If athletes in these younger age groups need to lose fat, caloric restriction should be utilized very carefully so as not to impair their growth. Emphasize increased energy expenditure through training rather than dieting. The suggestions in this chapter for reducing *fat* intake and not just *food* intake are also particularly useful for young athletes. No fat reduction eating program will ever be as spartan as the diet presented in Table 11.1.

In addition to ensuring adequate nutrition for growth, a slow rate of weight loss produces less mental strain. Because each pound of fat is equivalent to about 3,500 kilocalories (kcal), you can calculate the extent to which the caloric balance scales must be "tipped" to

Table 11.1
Wrestler's Diet for Losing Weight

Want to lose weight? Try this. You are guaranteed to lose weight (or your health).

Day	Meal	Menu
Monday	Breakfast Lunch Dinner	Weak tea 1 bouillon cube in ¼ cup of diluted water 1 pigeon thigh 3 oz prune juice (gargle only)
Tuesday	Breakfast Lunch Dinner	Scraped crumbs from burned toast 1 doughnut hole (without sugar) 1 glass of dehydrated water 2 grains of corn meal (broiled)
Wednesday	Breakfast Lunch Dinner	Boiled-out stains of tablecloth ½ doz poppy seeds Bee's knees and mosquito's knuckles sautéed in vinegar
Thursday	Breakfast Lunch Dinner	Shredded eggshell skins 1 belly button from a navel orange 3 eyes from Irish potato (diced)
Friday	Breakfast Lunch Dinner	2 lobster antennae 1 guppy fin Fillet of soft-shell crab claw
Saturday	Breakfast Lunch Dinner	4 chopped banana seeds Broiled butterfly liver Jellyfish vertebrae à la bookbinder
Sunday	Breakfast Lunch Dinner	Pickled hummingbird tongue Prime rib of tadpole Aroma of empty custard pie plate Tossed paprika and (1) clover leaf salad

Note. All meals should be eaten under a microscope to avoid extra portions.

achieve the desired fat loss by multiplying the number of pounds of desired fat loss by 3,500. Eric needs to lose 3 pounds of fat; by multiplying 3,500 by 3, we determine that he needs to tip his caloric balance scales by 10,500 kcal. Half these kilocalories should be accounted for through caloric restriction and half through in- creased physical activity, so Eric needs to re- strict his diet by 5,250 kcal and increase his activity by 5,250 kcal. We can now determine how long it will take Eric to accomplish his task. Theoretically, if you want Eric to lose a pound a week, just divide 3,500 into the total number of kilocalories (in Eric's case, 10,500).

If you want him to lose 2 pounds a week, divide the total by 7,000 kcal.

If Eric has 5 weeks until his first race, and if he loses 1 pound a week, he should be able to achieve his calculated optimal weight by the race. To do this, Eric must restrict his caloric intake by 1,750 kcal per week or 250 kcal per day. The feasibility of such a restriction can be evaluated considering Eric's present intake relative to his caloric requirement. This brings us to the fourth nutritional guideline.

Vary Requirements for Different Individuals

Individual caloric requirements are influenced by age, body surface area, growth rate, and physical activity level. There is no single specific requirement for everyone; each of us has different nutritional needs. The reason for the variability in caloric need is related to how we use the kilocalories that our diets provide as well as the type of food that we eat. Remember, we use food (a) to provide our bodies with needed vitamins, minerals, and other nutrients for the growth and repair of tissues; (b) to provide the energy to perform the automatic functions that sustain life (heart function, breathing, digestion, etc.); and (c) to provide the energy for moving our body parts, as during physical activity. As a general guideline, the Food and Nutrition Board (National Research Council, 1980) recommends the caloric levels in Table 11.2 for children.

These values, however, do not take individual variability and, more importantly, physical training into consideration. The youngster who participates in several hours of vigorous activity requires more kilocalories than a sedentary classmate. In addition, the type of activity makes a difference. As was shown in Table 3.2 (p. 24), the caloric costs of different activities vary significantly. Another factor that influences the energy requirement of an activity is the body weight of the person performing it. Most energy-cost charts are based on the energy costs of a 150-pound adult. A child who weighs only 110 pounds burns considerably fewer kilocalories for a given activity than an adult male who weighs 150 pounds. Charts that depict caloric cost values in kilocalories per minute per pound of body weight are the most accurate.

Nutrient density also influences the number of kilocalories that must be consumed. If most of the foods that a person eats have high nutrient density (i.e., have lots of vitamins and minerals per kilocalorie), the person needs to consume fewer calories to get all the nutrients the body requires.

Because of all of these difficulties with predicting an individual's caloric requirement, and because it is tedious and impractical to meticulously count calories all the time, do not actually make your athletes count their calories. Instead, focus on having them eat a balanced diet drawn from the four basic food groups.

Eat a Balanced Diet

A young athlete should obtain his or her daily caloric requirement from a balanced diet. A balanced diet is one that meets the body's nutrient and caloric needs. For instance, it is possible to get the necessary number of kilocalories to meet the calorie needs by eating nothing but cupcakes. Such a diet, however, does not supply all the essential amino acids nor the appropriate vitamins and minerals. As you can see in Table 11.3, most of the protein, iron, and vitamin A in a cupcake come from the eggs. Potassium, thiamine, and riboflavin come from the eggs and the milk. A glass of skim milk, a piece of toast, and a poached egg

Table 11.2
Recommended Caloric Intake Levels for Children

Gender	Age	Number of kcal/day
Boys and girls	1-3	1,300
	3-6	1,600
	6-9	2,100
Boys	9-12	2,400
	12-15	3,000
	15-18	3,400
Girls	9-12	2,200
	12-15	2,500
	15-18	2,300

Table 11.3

Comparison of Nutrient Value of Cupcakes, Eggs, and Skim Milk

One pound of:	Food energy (kcal)	Protein (g)	Carbohydrate (g)	Calcium (mg)	Phosphorus (mg)	Iron (mg)	Sodium (mg)	Potassium (mg)	Vitamin A (IU)	Thiamine (mg)	Riboflavin (mg)	Niacin (mg)	Vitamin C (mg)
Cupcake mix made with eggs, milk, and chocolate icing	1,624	20.4	268.5	590	894	3.6	1,520	531	770	0.16	0.49	1.0	trace
Eggs	739	58.5	4.1	245	930	10.4	553	585	5,350	0.48	1.35	0.3	0
Skim milk	163	16.3	23.1	549	431	0.2	236	658	20	0.16	0.80	0.3	5

has about the same number of kilocalories as two cupcakes but much more nutrition.

Having your athletes eat selections from the four basic food groups helps to ensure a balanced diet. The four basic groups and the recommended portions of each were presented in Table 3.3 (p. 25). Additional information on evaluating the balanced diet is provided later in this chapter.

Drink Water

Daily water consumption is an absolute must. As we have emphasized over and over, weight loss should come from the fat stores, the body's true excess weight, and not the body's vital water supply. *Never* allow your athletes to go without water (see Figure 11.5).

WEIGHT LOSS STEPS

Now that you know the six guidelines for losing fat weight, you are ready to learn how to implement a fat loss program. The steps for doing this are presented next.

Weight Loss Steps

Step 1: Determine body composition
Step 2: Establish fat loss goals
Step 3: Evaluate dietary habits
Step 4: Avoid crash diets
Step 5: Eat several times a day
Step 6: Drink water
Step 7: Train systematically
Step 8: Utilize behavior modification techniques
Step 9: Monitor performance
Step 10: Maintain optimal weight

Determine Body Composition

Determine the athlete's body composition 6 to 8 weeks prior to the season. Use this information to predict the athlete's optimal body weight. By completing the procedures described in chapter 2, you can show your athletes how much of their body weight is made up of fat, and you can give them individualized fat loss goals. Remember, you must not let your athletes get carried away and try to reach 0% fat. In doing so, they will jeopardize not only their athletic careers but their physical health as well. All human beings need some body fat!

Establish Fat Loss Goals

Present each athlete's fat loss goals in fat loss timetables. These tables can serve as impor-

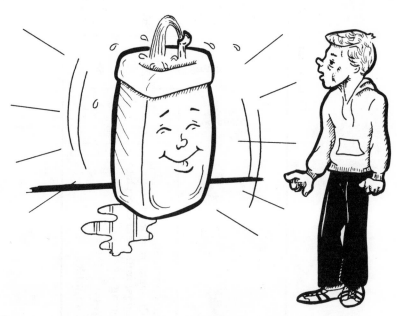

Figure 11.5.   Athletes and water fountains should become good friends.

tant feedback devices for the athlete as he or she engages in a fat loss program. Evaluating body composition and predicting optimal weight is relatively easy, but actually getting the athlete to make the necessary training and lifestyle changes to reach and maintain his or her optimal percent fat is much more difficult. To help with this, do not pressure your athletes to reach their optimal weights quickly and do *not* use the word *diet*. Instead, encourage athletes to view the fat control process as a valuable part of life in general, not just a short-term fix.

A sample fat loss timetable is illustrated in Figure 11.6. In it, Selma, a 157-pound female high school basketball player, has made a graph with body weight on the left side and time in weeks on the bottom. She has about 6 weeks before the season starts, so her coach has suggested that she put 6 weeks on the bottom line of the graph. Because she has 12 pounds of fat to lose, she is within the safety range of 2 pounds per week. If Selma had more weight to lose, the time line at the bottom of the graph would be extended, and she would continue to work on fat reduction even after the season started.

After making the graph, Selma should plot her starting weight (157 pounds) and her optimum weight (145 pounds) and connect these two points with a straight line. This is a "goal line" and shows that Selma has a weekly goal of 2 pounds of fat loss each week. Two times a week, on the same days and at about the same time, Selma should weigh herself and record the weight on the fat loss chart. If these weight plot points fall below the goal line, it indicates that she is losing weight too rapidly. This means that she is probably losing lean or muscle tissue as well as fat stores, and she

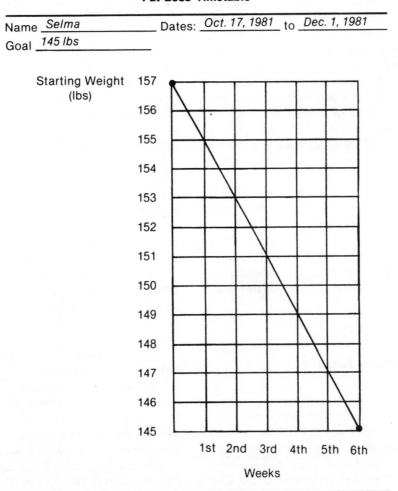

Fat Loss Timetable

Name _Selma_   Dates: _Oct. 17, 1981_ to _Dec. 1, 1981_
Goal _145 lbs_

Figure 11.6. Selma plotted her fat loss goals on a timetable.

must therefore be discouraged from becoming overzealous about losing weight. If, on the other hand, Selma's weight plot points are above the goal line, her fat reduction may not be on schedule. We use the word *may* because there are alternative explanations for a lack of weight loss. Of course the most obvious is that she has not made eating changes or is not adhering to the training schedule, so fat has not been lost. A second possible explanation is that lean weight gains as a result of training are offsetting her fat losses. It is also possible that weight due to increases in the storage of glycogen and increases in blood volume may account for weight gains at the beginning of training programs (Convertino, Brook, Keil, Bernauer, & Greenleaf, 1980). A weekly record of skinfold thickness will help you determine the explanation for a lack of decrease in body weight.

You may also find a chart for tracking skinfold thickness useful. The chart should be similar to the fat loss timetable in providing a place for recording weekly changes in skinfold thickness that occur with fat loss. It differs from the fat loss timetable in that it does not have a goal line. As fat is lost, one of the storage sites just beneath the skin should decrease in size; therefore decreases in fat weight should be reflected in decreases in skinfold thickness. However, we do not know the exact rate at which skinfold thickness decreases with fat loss. Consequently a goal line cannot be drawn.

As discussed in chapter 2 the subscapular and calf skinfolds are particularly good sites for tracking fat loss, so you should construct a graph for each of these skinfold sites. Over the course of the weight loss period the thickness of the fat at both of these sites should decrease if the athlete is losing fat and not lean tissue.

Evaluate Dietary Habits

Have athletes evaluate their present nutritional habits and practices by completing the Diet Habit Survey (Connor & Connor, 1986). A copy of this survey is found in Appendix B. This survey was developed as a tool for determining whether people eat balanced diets. The responses to the questions in each section of the survey help athletes see if they are selecting foods from the four basic food groups. In addition, the survey evaluates the types of food within each food group athletes choose to eat. Athletes will receive better scores if they select low-fat rather than high-fat foods.

Have your athletes respond to the questions in the eight sections of the survey. These sections are meat, fish, and poultry; dairy products and eggs; fats and oils; grains, beans, fruits, and vegetables; sweets, snacks, and beverages; salt; restaurant choices; and overall eating style. Responses are tabulated and interpreted by adding the scores from each question in a section. These total scores are then recorded in the column on the far right on the appropriate assessment chart. There are two assessment charts in Appendix B—one for women and children, the other for men and teens.

The assessment chart on page 162, for men and teens, was selected for Selma because she is a teenage basketball player. The total score for each section has been recorded in the column entitled "Selma's Score." Once the section total scores have been recorded they can be totaled, and the interpretation process begins.

Although completing of the Diet Habit Survey requires some time, it is time well spent. In completing the survey, an athlete is taking an active role in determining his or her own destiny. The survey score provides a tool for evaluating the athlete's eating habits. If these habits are less than optimal, which is typical for most Americans, the survey also serves as a guide for identifying nutritional goals for the athlete. For example, the column on the assessment form entitled "Present American diet" lists the scores that Selma would probably achieve if she ate what most Americans presently eat. Most Americans eat high-fat foods that do not provide the carbohydrates needed for training or optimal weight maintenance. The three columns labeled "Phase I," "Phase II," and "Phase III" present progressively better dietary habits.

The goal for optimal nutrition is for the athlete to score at the Phase III level in all survey categories. If the athlete's scores fall within this phase, he or she is eating a diet that is providing lots of carbohydrates rich in vitamins and minerals. More specifically, at the Phase III level the diet is 65% carbohydrate, 15% protein, and only 20% fat. In other words, the athlete is eating a balanced diet.

Assessment of the Diet Habit Survey Scores for 2,800 Calories

Men/Teens

Food group	Present American diet	The New American Diet Phase			Selma's score
		I	II	III	
Meat, fish, and poultry	< 11	11-12	15-17	20-24	17
Dairy products and eggs	< 23	23-26	29-32	31-35	26
Fats and oils	< 13	13-15	18-20	21-24	16
Grains, beans, fruits, and vegetables	< 70	70-91	98-123	129-160	75
Sweets, snacks, and beverages	< 18	18	24-28	29-30	25
Salt	< 14	14-16	20	24-25	15
Restaurant choices	< 15	15-35	40-60	65-75	35
Overall eating style	< 6	6	8	10	6
Total	<147	170-219	252-308	329-383	215

These total scores correspond to a diet with the following nutrient composition:

Cholesterol, mg/day	500	<350	<220	<140	_____
Saturated fat, % kcal	14	10	8	5	_____
Fats, % kcal	40	35	25	20	_____
Carbohydrates, % kcal	45	50	60	65	_____
Protein, % kcal	15	15	15	15	_____
Sodium, mg/day	>4,025	4,025	3,220	2,415	_____
Potassium, mg/day	<3,549	3,549	5,460	5,460	_____

Note. From *The New American Diet* by S.L. Connor and W.E. Connor, 1986, New York: Simon & Schuster. Copyright 1986 by Sonja L. Connor, M.S., R.D. and William E. Connor, M.D. Reprinted by permission of Simon and Schuster, Inc.

As you see from Selma's scores on the Diet Habit Survey assessment form (see the column on the far right), Selma has considerable room for improvement in her diet. She is at Phase I in five of the eight categories and her total score of 215 places her dietary habits at the Phase I level. Though her ultimate goal should be to reach Phase III, she can begin this process by making dietary changes so that she can progress to Phase II. Of all the food groups, the grains, beans, fruits, and vegetables group has the most potential for adding points to her score. By incorporating more of these food choices into her diet she will get more nutrients and also begin to fulfill the objective of eating a high-carbohydrate diet. Therefore, Selma's number-one goal should be to increase her score in the grains, beans, fruits, and vegetables category. If this number-one goal is coupled with efforts to increase her score in the dairy products and eggs category as well as the fat and oils category, Selma will easily be able to decrease her caloric intake and lose the necessary body fat by substituting high-carbohydrate, low-fat foods for the high-fat foods she is currently eating. Some specific suggestions for helping Selma make these changes include the following:

- Eat more fresh fruits, especially for snacks; substitute fruit snacks for chocolate, potato chips, french fries, corn chips, and high-fat cookies.
- Eat more vegetables (without sauces).
- Eat baked potatoes, macaroni, or rice (served without fats or oils).
- Reduce your servings of meat; when you do eat meat, select lean red meats, and serve chicken and turkey sandwiches without cheese or mayonnaise.
- Have salads for lunch; select low-fat dressings.

- Substitute low-fat cheese for high-fat cheese.
- Eat fewer egg yolks.

You can develop these types of suggestions for your athletes by looking back at the specific questions in the survey. For example, if in response to the second question in the meat, fish, and poultry section (p. 152) the athlete has indicated that his or her typical lunch consists of cheeseburgers and typical cheese or egg dishes, that athlete scores only one point. Suggest that the athlete start choosing chicken, turkey, or tuna sandwiches without mayo. As you can see, these choices will result in higher scores on the diet survey.

In addition to making some changes in her eating habits, Selma should also train so that her caloric needs stay elevated (Donahoe, Lin, Kirschenbaum, & Keesey, 1984). A high-carbohydrate diet helps provide her with the energy necessary to maintain her training schedule.

Avoid Crash Diets

Neither the goal of achieving Phase III on the Diet Habit Survey nor the goal of achieving optimal performance may be realized by severely restricting caloric consumption. Instead, the athlete's objective should be to select high-nutrient-density foods—foods that are loaded with vitamins and minerals relative to the number of calories. Such a diet is high in carbohydrates. Contrary to popular belief, carbohydrates are not fattening. In fact, quite the reverse is true. It is more difficult for the body to store carbohydrates as fat than to store dietary fat as fat in the adipose cells of the body (Acheson, Flatt, & Jequier, 1982; Acheson, Schutz, Bessard, Ravussin, & Jequier, 1984).

Occasionally a doctor will prescribe a very low-calorie diet, but in such cases vitamin and mineral supplements are also prescribed. Also remember that individuals on these types of diets are not training to enhance their performance potential as athletes. Never recommend such a stringent diet regime.

Eat Several Times a Day

Encourage athletes never to skip meals and to spread out the calories they consume. It has been shown that missing breakfast can reduce an individual's effectiveness by 25%, which can make it hard for young athletes to do their schoolwork (see Figure 11.7). Athletes trying to reduce weight may eat five times a day—three meals and two snacks. "Snacks," however, should consist of protein or carbohydrate rather than fat and junk foods. Eating five times a day spreads out caloric intake over the whole day, keeping the athlete's appetite more satisfied. With this strategy, blood sugar levels are more likely to be stable. In addition, research has demonstrated that the gastrointestinal tract is less efficient if food intake is spread out over five or six meals, meaning that fewer kilocalories are absorbed into the bloodstream. If only one meal is consumed, the gastrointestinal tract is very efficient in extracting all available kilocalories (La Veille & Romsos, 1974).

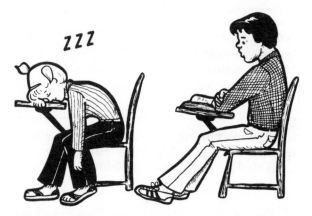

Figure 11.7. Missing breakfast can make students sleepy and impair their schoolwork.

There is also support for the fact that there is an increase in the thermic effect of exercise if the athlete is consuming meals on a regular basis. This means that more calories are burned when the athlete is exercising and eating rather than exercising and fasting (Segal & Gutin, 1983).

Drink Water

Athletes should drink one quart of water for every 1,000 kilocalories eaten. Water, which has no caloric value, is one of the most important elements of the weight loss program. Therefore, athletes should cultivate good water-drinking habits.

Train Systematically

Too often, coaches require their athletes to play their way into condition for their sport. This does not optimally develop the body's energy-producing systems nor does it help the athlete burn excess fat stores. A systematic approach to training results in a fitter athlete and a potentially better performer. A fitter individual also better utilizes fat as a fuel (Despres, Bouchard, Savard, Tremblay, Marcotte, and Theriault, 1984).

Utilize Behavior Modification Techniques

Achieving optimal weight goals depends on the athlete changing dietary and training habits. In other words, your athletes will need to modify their eating and exercising behaviors. Because a considerable degree of motivation is necessary to initiate and maintain new behaviors, knowledge of motivational strategies and other aspects of the psychological aspects of weight loss are also important. Psychologists have suggested a number of "tricks" to help people trying to lose weight. Many of these tricks, or modifications of them, are valuable to athletes.

For example, to help keep athletes motivated, compiling a list of physical and psychological hazards associated with not losing excess fat weight can help athletes avoid resorting to the "roller-coaster approach" to making weight (see Figure 11.8). Some of these hazards include the following:

- It causes ups and downs in energy levels.
- On some days training seems almost impossibly difficult.
- Athletes become less resistant to infections and get sick, preventing them from being able to train.
- A "down" feeling that can be associated with dips in blood glucose level often results from crash dieting.
- It is difficult to maintain the positive self-image essential for quality training and practice to take place (see Figure 11.9).
- A person who feels tired and irritable responds to family and friends differently (see Figure 11.10).
- Being sleepy all the time can make schoolwork suffer.

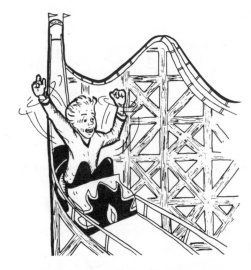

Figure 11.8. The roller-coaster approach to making weight must be avoided; instead, athletes should pursue long-term fat control programs.

Motivation can also be enhanced by using incentives and rewards. Parents and coaches in particular can play an important role in this process. Using the weight and skinfold charts as a record of achieved goals, parents and coaches can acknowledge the realization of each goal with many types of rewards, including

- doing something special with the family or a friend (other than eating);
- treating the athlete to an extra hour of sleep on Saturday mornings;
- allowing the athlete to choose a favorite program on the family television;
- going on a shopping trip for a needed or desired object (e.g., clothes, records, or books); or
- excusing the athlete from a specific chore on a given day (like washing dishes or taking out trash).

These are only a few of the ideas that psychologists have proposed. For additional ideas, you may wish to obtain some of the books listed on page 109 that explore in more detail behavior modification to aid with weight loss.

Monitor Performance

Fat loss and changes in skinfold thickness reinforce the achievement of weight loss goals, but neither you nor your athletes should lose sight of the fact that the true purpose for

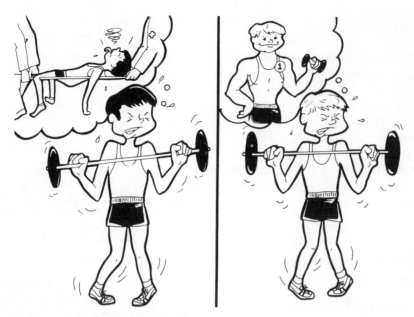

Figure 11.9. Athletes' self-confidence is affected by what they eat and don't eat. If an athlete's body is suffering from a crash diet, self-concept is likely to suffer as well.

the fat loss is improved performance. Consequently, if performance ability is not improving, the ultimate objective is not being achieved. Utilize objective criteria and good judgment to determine if athletes are losing weight properly. If you monitor the performance of your athletes so that you can answer the following questions, you will be able to tell if the fat loss is actually helping your athletes.

- Is the athlete maintaining muscular strength or is it deteriorating? This can be determined by periodically testing the athlete's strength.
- Is the athlete maintaining speed and quickness? Again, actual measurement and tracking of training progress allows you to answer this question and evaluate the success of the fat loss and training program.
- Does the athlete appear to "wear down" at the end of practice, games, or matches?
- Does the athlete appear lethargic and inattentive in classes, at practice, or at home?
- Has the athlete demonstrated a marked change in personality or disposition during the weight loss period? Some athletes experience severe psychological disturbances that result in eating disorders. Chapter 12 specifically addresses this important issue.

Maintain Optimal Weight

Once an athlete has reached the optimal weight, ensure that the weight is maintained. You can help athletes by providing frequent weigh-ins so that their weights do not "bounce" up and down. If you allow great fluctuation, your athletes will probably use crash diets and dehydration to control their weight.

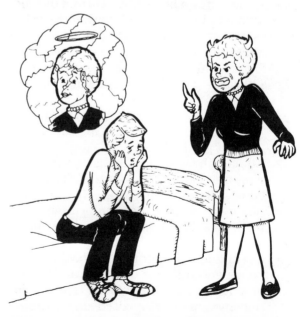

Figure 11.10. Crash dieters frequently feel that their loved ones have "turned" on them.

Book	Authors	Publisher
Thin and Fit: Your Personal Lifestyle	Dusek, D.	Wadsworth, Belmont, CA
Slim Chance in a Fat World: Behavioral Control of Obesity	Stuart, R.B., & Davis, B.	Research Press, Champaign, IL
How to Lower Your Fat Thermostat	Remington, D.W., Fisher, A.G., & Parent, E.A.	Vitality House International Provo, UT

This exposes them to at least three physiological disadvantages. First, they will deplete the carbohydrate stores in their muscles if they undergo 24 to 48 hours of semistarvation. These stores constitute the immediate source of explosive energy athletes need. Second, the chemical and water balance in the blood and fluids around the cells will be upset. This also detracts from performance efficiency. Third, the roller-coaster approach to making weight prevents the body from acclimatizing and stabilizing. Athletes' vitality is lowered, weakness sets in, and athletes become more susceptible to colds and infection (National Dairy Council, 1985).

As you can see, helping athletes to maintain their ideal weight throughout the season provides them with some nutritional conditioning. In fact, you are helping athletes develop sound lifelong dietary habits.

SUMMARY AND RECOMMENDATIONS

Among the many factors that influence the performance potential of your athletes are body composition, dietary habits, and training habits. Now that you understand how and why these factors are important, you need to put this knowledge to use by helping your athletes lose fat weight sensibly. This can be best accomplished if you take the following steps:

1. Determine the body composition of your athletes 6 to 8 weeks prior to the season, and use this information to predict an optimum weight range for each athlete.

2. Set up recording forms for tracking fat loss and changes in skinfold thickness. This will help you emphasize to your athletes that body composition, rather than just scale weight, is important. Use these charts to identify athletes who are losing weight too rapidly, perhaps through crash dieting.

3. Have your athletes complete the Diet Habit Survey so you can identify the specific eating behaviors each athlete needs to alter.

4. Give athletes specific suggestions for changing their eating habits. These suggestions can be derived from the question section of the Diet Habit Survey.

5. Encourage your athletes never to skip meals and to spread out the calories consumed. (Remember, snacks should be high in protein or carbohydrates; they should not be junk foods.)

6. Ensure that athletes replace the fluids lost during practice and training sessions. This will help teach them good water-drinking habits.

7. Implement systematic training sessions to enhance the capabilities of the energy systems used in your particular sport and to provide athletes with a mechanism for increasing their caloric expenditure.

8. Utilize behavior modification techniques to help maintain motivation during the weight loss period.

9. Monitor performance during the fat loss period so you can evaluate the efficacy of the fat loss program.

10. Continue to emphasize the importance of high-carbohydrate, low-fat food choices

even after athletes achieve their optimal weights. This ensures that your athletes always have the energy to train hard and recover from the training.

Although the focus of this chapter has been on losing fat weight, all the nutritional guidelines and specific steps presented are appropriate for all athletes. Not only will these strategies help achieve optimal weight, they will also facilitate energy management and help your athletes develop healthy eating habits to serve them well as they grow into adulthood.

Chapter 12
Eating Disorders in Athletes

Throughout this book we have emphasized the importance of optimal weight for optimal performance. As the world of sport and performance emphasizes optimizing lean weight and getting rid of fat, society's "ideal" female body grows progressively thinner. Unfortunately, however, the average *real* American woman is getting fatter. This paradoxical situation places a great deal of pressure on women; the media and other institutions have created an image that equates success and beauty with thinness. This was not the case two decades ago. For example, investigators studying *Playboy* magazine centerfolds from 1959 to 1978 found that the models' average weight in relation to height had declined by 8% over those two decades. This period has also seen a significant increase in eating disorders. It has been speculated that societal and cultural pressures toward thinness have resulted in increased incidence of abnormal eating behaviors.

The findings of a recent Gallup poll revealed that two million Americans suffer from eating disorders, with the highest incidence among teenage girls. It has been estimated that 16% of high school-age girls and 20% of college-age women have either anorexia nervosa or bulimia. *Anorexia nervosa* is an illness characterized by the relentless pursuit of thinness, even to the point of death by starvation. *Bulimia* is characterized by repeated eating binges (gorging oneself with food) and then purging the body of the food either by vomiting, abusing laxatives or diuretics, or fasting. If untreated, either can lead to serious physical and behavioral consequences, in some cases causing death.

WHY DO ATHLETES DEVELOP EATING DISORDERS?

As previously stated, the exact cause of eating disorders is unknown, but girls and women, as well as some men involved in weight-control sports and activities, appear to be at increased risk. As we pointed out in chapters 1 and 2, optimal body weight gives the performer a distinct edge in competition. An increased strength-to-weight ratio can enhance gymnastic performance. Lower body-fat levels in endurance athletes result in improved aerobic power and speed. When the stressors of adolescence and those associated with highly competitive sports are combined with too much emphasis on leanness or an emphasis on inappropriate weight control techniques, the resultant emotional and physical pressure can become enormous. This pressure, according to some authorities, may cause an athlete to cross the fine line between dieting to achieve an appropriate competition weight and total obsession with body weight and food.

Sport-Specific Reasons

Participants in some high-risk sports are faced with another dilemma in that their training activities, which include only brief periods of low- to high-level activity, are too intermittent to have much effect on either maximal aerobic power or calorie expenditure. Because they do not burn many calories, they do not have large caloric needs. Therefore, in an effort to comply with rigorous body size or weight requirements, gymnasts, ballet dancers, and wrestlers may resort to caloric restriction and sometimes aberrant eating behaviors.

Susceptible Athletes

One theory for explaining the relatively high incidence of eating disorders among female athletes suggests that weight control pressures drive certain athletes to eating disorders. Another theory maintains that individuals with personalities that make them susceptible to eating disorders are attracted to the weight control sports. In fact, the initial discipline and dedication the athlete shows in controlling weight may make the individual successful in the sport or activity at first. Inevitably, though, an untreated eating disorder can destroy the athlete's career and can even take his or her life.

It is imperative that coaches be alert to the signs and symptoms of eating disorders. This is not to say that coaches should make medical diagnoses, but you are in an excellent position to observe early signs of disorder and direct athletes to professional help. It is no easy task to spot early problems. However, the difficulty of identifying anorexia nervosa and bulimia in high-level athletes, who are required to be lean and are therefore justifiably attentive to controlling their weight, cannot be overemphasized. Indeed, it has been suggested that success in athletic endeavors, as well as in weight control, depends on a certain degree of obsession. It is a mistake to assume that dieting behavior or weight preoccupation alone signifies an eating disorder. In fact, specific criteria must be met for the diagnosis of both anorexia nervosa and bulimia.

IDENTIFYING ANOREXIA NERVOSA

Anorexia nervosa is a clinical syndrome of self-induced starvation characterized by a voluntary refusal to eat due to an intense fear of fatness and a disturbed perception of body image. One to three percent of American girls 12 to 18 years of age will develop anorexia nervosa to some degree. Although 90% of anorexics are adolescent or young females, about 5% to 10% are males, usually involved in weight-conscious sports such as wrestling.

Physical Signs and Symptoms

Many of the changes that signal a potential problem with anorexia nervosa are linked to inadequate caloric intake. As a coach, you should recognize several physical signs.

Weight Loss

Extreme weight loss, usually amounting to more than 25% of the original body weight, occurs during the course of the disease. Using the body weight and skinfold thickness goal charts described in chapter 11 can help you detect excess weight loss in your athletes.

Amenorrhea

Amenorrhea (absent or irregular menstrual cycles) is thought to be the result of low body fat, intense exercise, low circulating estrogen levels, and possibly emotional stress. Not every amenorrheic athlete has an eating disorder, but every amenorrheic athlete should be encouraged to pay special attention to getting adequate nutrients (see chapter 8).

Low Metabolism

Low body temperature, heart rate, and blood pressure are probably the result of a decreased metabolic rate. Anorexic athletes may complain of being cold or may have icy hands and feet even when other people around them are warm. Orthostatic hypotension, or a drop in blood pressure when the athlete gets up quickly, may result in brief fainting or blackout episodes.

Skin Changes

The skin of an anorexic athlete may have a dry, inelastic appearance and a yellowish hue. A wrinkled and sunken face may make the individual look old. Lanugo, or soft fine hair, often covers the skin of the arms and face. Hair loss and brittle, broken nails may be the result of a low protein intake and are especially evident in athletes who are also strict vegetarians.

Constipation

Constipation may also be a problem. Due to the low food intake, fiber in the anorexic's diet is also low, and the movement of the intestine is decreased. This lack of normal movement of food through the intestine translates into fewer bowel movements and may cause the athlete to complain of abdominal pain.

Abnormal Sleep Patterns

Insomnia and other abnormal sleep patterns frequently occur, thought to be the result of abnormal brain function due to low nutrient intake. The athlete may be unable to concentrate on training or schoolwork as a result of sleep deprivation.

Psychological Signs

In addition to the physical signs that suggest anorexia nervosa, there are a number of psychological signs that coaches should watch for. Again, the presence of these traits or attributes does not necessarily mean that the athlete actually has anorexia nervosa. The diagnosis should be left to the professionals.

Body Image Problems

The anorexic athlete relentlessly pursues thinness. Even when emaciated, anorexics insist they are too fat and resist any suggestion to the contrary. They simply do not have a realistic picture of their bodies. Consequently, anorexics are continually driven to starve themselves.

Emotionally Suppressed

Anorexic athletes may be out of touch with their emotions and unable to express anger. Some authorities believe that anorexics might use their eating disorders as a vehicle for expressing rage or resentment. Sometimes athletes who believe they are not being fairly recognized for their performance or ability believe that this recognition can be achieved through the attainment of very low body fat. In fact, anorexic athletes often say to themselves, "If I can't be the best, at least I can be the thinnest."

Perfectionism

Obedient and cooperative, anorexic athletes typically come from white, upper-middle-class families that emphasize high achievement and attractive physical appearance. The anorexic tends to be successful academically and a good athlete. Coaches find these athletes to be highly motivated players, rarely missing practice and never arguing with coaching decisions. In striving for perfection and approval, the anorexic begins dieting to lose a few pounds; after the initial target weight has been reached, however, dieting does not stop.

Low Self-Esteem and Fear of Growing Up

Feelings of worthlessness or hopelessness may plague anorexic athletes, despite a history of achievement in sports and academics. They do not accept praise easily.

The body fat normally deposited during the maturational processes associated with adolescence may be viewed as an unwanted harbinger of adulthood. Because the decreased independence and responsibility that comes with adulthood may be frightening, some authorities speculate that a fear of independence may motivate the anorexic athlete to starve in an attempt to delay or prevent puberty. In other words, by keeping a childlike body, the anorexic believes the problems of growing up can be avoided.

Lack of Control

A sense of lack of control may dominate the anorexic athlete. Families of these individuals have a low tolerance for conflict and are highly controlling. The pursuit of thinness is regarded as the anorexic's struggle to exert control and self-direction. A highly controlling or dominating coach may further compound this problem. Therefore, coaches need to be very careful when discussing fat loss targets. The athlete's goal should be the adoption of a well-balanced high-carbohydrate, low-fat diet, not just fat loss in itself.

Behavioral Signs

Behavioral signs constitute still another way that alert coaches may see potential indicators of anorexia nervosa. Coaches work on a day-to-day basis with athletes and are therefore in an excellent position to observe behavioral tendencies.

Denial

Anorexic athletes deny hunger and thinness and stubbornly refuse to eat, although hunger is always present. They may not eat the pregame meal with the rest of the team, insisting that they are too nervous. If the team goes out to eat after the game or competition, the anorexic athlete may sip a diet soda while the rest of the team eats a meal, stating that it is still too soon to eat, and insisting that he or she will eat something at home, although this is rarely the truth. Anorexia means "loss of appetite;" however, most anorexics do not experience a true loss of appetite until late in starvation. Early on, they simply control their fierce hunger.

Very Low Calorie Intakes

Even the most active anorexic athletes eat only 300 to 1,100 calories per day. Anorexics hide food, hoard food, and avoid social situations or team parties where they may feel pressured or tempted to eat. However, anorexics often develop a keen interest in cooking and grocery shopping. Poring over cookbooks and nutrition texts, they become experts in the areas of diet and nutrition. They are the athletes that teammates seek out for information on the caloric content of foods.

Rituals

The anorexic athlete may adopt ritualistic food behaviors such as cutting food into small portions, eating foods in a specific order, pushing food around the plate, or blotting meats with a paper towel to remove every trace of fat.

They are also ritualistic in their exercise programs. Even when nearing exhaustion, the anorexic athlete may engage in "extra" training sessions that tend to be solitary and obsessive in nature. For example, such an athlete might perform a preplanned set of exercises with a given number in each set (100 pushups, 100 sit-ups) daily in addition to the training program you plan for the athlete.

As their disease progresses, anorexic athletes may become increasingly withdrawn. Breaking off relationships with teammates and friends, they may rarely laugh or smile. They usually do not date and are sexually inactive.

IDENTIFYING BULIMIA

Bulimia is defined as recurrent episodes of rapid, uncontrollable ingestion of large amounts of food in a short period of time, usually followed by purging either by forced vomiting, abuse of laxatives or diuretics, or both. The purging techniques are used to decrease possible weight gain, relieve fullness, and restore the individual's sense of control.

Although the actual incidence of bulimia has not been clearly established, it is thought that 5% to 15% of high school-age girls and 19% to 20% of college-age women are affected. Bulimia is suspected to be more prevalent among males than anorexia nervosa, though more difficult to detect.

Physical Signs and Symptoms

The binging and purging cycles associated with bulimia have slightly different effects on the body than the starvation practice associated with anorexia nervosa. Again, the observant coach should be alert to these signs to help the athlete get professional help if necessary.

Normal Body Size

Anorexics look emaciated, but bulimics cannot be identified by appearance alone. A bulimic athlete may be thin, normal weight, or overweight. Frequent weight fluctuations of 10 pounds or more in a bulimic athlete are a function of binging and the subsequent purging of food. Again, the tables for recording weights and skinfold measurements presented in chapter 11 should be helpful in alerting you to unusual weight loss or weight gain patterns.

Impaired Performance

Dehydration, worsening athletic performance, and fainting episodes are caused by electrolyte disturbances resulting from frequent vomiting or laxative or diuretic abuse. On the night before the state track championships, one top high school 3,000-meter runner was so anxious that she ate an entire gallon of ice cream and purged by vomiting. At the meet the next day, she added 30 seconds to her usual time and lost the state title simply because she ran out of energy during the last lap.

Any athlete who passes out should be checked by the team physician for further physical signs of bulimia or other serious health problems. The team physician may spot an irregular heartbeat, which again is the result of electrolyte disturbances.

Throat and Dental Problems

An irritated esophagus and complaints of frequent sore throats in a bulimic athlete may be due to the exposure of these soft tissues to the harsh secretions of the stomach during vomiting.

Tooth erosion occurs when the acidic substances from the stomach make contact with the teeth. In fact, it is often the athlete's dentist who first diagnoses bulimia. And swollen parotid glands caused by excessive saliva production from vomiting create a chipmunk-like face in even a slender athlete.

Psychological Signs

Coaches who are attentive to the personalities, moods, and feelings of their athletes have the best chance of being able to identify psychological signs that may signify bulimia.

Fear of Fat

The relentless pursuit of thinness and an overriding awareness that their eating pattern is abnormal are hallmarks of bulimics. Yet bulimics believe they are powerless to stop. So they continue the binge-purge cycle and try to keep it a secret. Initially these athletes may be successful competitors because they can maintain the desired body weight and still train effectively. Eventually, however, their physical performance suffers as the impact of the purging accumulates.

Mood Swings

Bulimic athletes are susceptible to tremendous mood swings. They may be euphoric one minute, angry or sullen the next. They are often extreme personalities and may even entertain thoughts of suicide. Feelings of guilt and self-deprecation may trigger a binge or may follow a period of binge eating and will be relieved only by purging. There may be a link between depression and bulimia. If so, the treatment of depression may also relieve bulimic behavior.

Behavioral Signs

Although bulimics tend to be very secretive about binging and purging, there are some subtle indicators. You will not detect these behavioral indicators on the field or court or in the gym, but if you are observant, you may pick up hints by observing the athletes before and after practice.

Binge Eating and Purging

Recurrent episodes of binge eating with the intent of purging later can happen as often as 20 times a day. Bulimic athletes may consume 3,000 to 20,000 calories at a time, and some reports say they spend as much as $250 a week to support their behavior. Shoplifting groceries and other items or hoarding secret caches of food are not uncommon. Binging is also done in secret. Bulimics may describe their feelings during such an episode as hypnotic or trance-like.

Self-induced vomiting is the most common purging technique employed by the bulimic athlete to regain the control lost during a binge. Be alert to the smell of vomit in the gym restroom or to an athlete who habitually excuses himself or herself after a meal.

Aggressive Behavior

Impulsive behavior is more common in bulimia than in anorexia nervosa. Bulimics are often intolerant of frustration and may disrupt training sessions or competition with emotional outbursts. Alcohol and drug abuse may also be a problem for these athletes.

DISTINGUISHING EATING DISORDERS

There is some confusion and controversy regarding whether bulimia and anorexia nervosa are separate, mutually exclusive syndromes or overlapping disorders. Some anorexic athletes engage in purging behavior, and some bulimic patients are emaciated or anorexic in appearance. According to the diagnostic criteria of the American Psychiatric Association, bulimia is limited to individuals who are at or above normal weight. Nevertheless, about 30% to 50% of patients with anorexia nervosa will later develop symptoms of bulimia. So if you know that one of your athletes has a history of anorexia nervosa, be alert to the development of any signs of bulimia. If you suspect there is a problem, *identifying which eating disorder your athlete has is not as important as seeking immediate professional help.*

EFFECTS OF EATING DISORDERS UPON PERFORMANCE

In chapter 5 we compared the trained human body to a high-performance sports car. We made this comparison because we believe that athletes should be concerned with optimizing their bodies' performance just as the owner of the sports car tries to optimize the car's performance. One essential strategy for ensuring a car's performance is to fill it with high-quality fuel. Similarly, the purpose of the dietary strategies presented in this book is to help athletes select the best possible foods to fuel their bodies. By not eating appropriately, the athlete with an eating disorder sabotages performance potential just as surely as does the owner of a high-performance car who uses cheap, low-quality fuel. In fact, the physiologic consequences of fasting, crash dieting, self-induced vomiting, and taking laxatives and diuretics at the very least impair strength, endurance, and reaction time and in all likelihood endanger the athlete's health.

Glycogen Depletion

Anorexic athletes who starve themselves or bulimics who utilize purging techniques can-not replace muscle glycogen stores that have been depleted during physical activity. Such a depletion is strongly related to physical exhaustion. Over time, their ability to generate force and strength will be impaired because muscle fibers are depleted of glycogen, and movement control or movement correction are negatively influenced. Thus, depleted athletes may be unable to prevent themselves from sustaining injuries.

Athletes with eating disorders may also have low nutrient stores and therefore may be unable to heal quickly once an injury has occurred. Anorexic female athletes who lose their normal menstrual cycles (the condition known as amenorrhea) risk bone density loss as well. Decreased bone mass translates into increased bone fragility and a greater likelihood for stress fractures. In fact, some researchers have shown that amenorrheic athletes may be at a greater risk for injuries besides just those related to bone density.

Metabolic Disruptions and Sudden Death

Starvation results in the breakdown of lean body tissue or muscle mass, including the heart muscle. Vomiting and laxative or diuretic abuse can also cause severe electrolyte disturbances resulting in irregular heartbeats. Thus, both anorexic and bulimic athletes risk sudden death from cardiac arrest on the playing field.

Decreased Fat-Free Weight

The constant weight fluctuations in bulimic individuals and the progressive and extreme loss of body weight in anorexic athletes have similar undesirable effects on body composition. When a person eats very few calories (less than 1,000), the body has to turn to its own tissues for fuel. When this occurs, less than 50% of that fuel comes from the body's fat stores; the rest is drawn from muscle. Therefore, the athlete loses lean weight. If weight is rapidly regained, as might occur with a bulimic athlete, the new weight will be predominantly fat weight. In this way, severe weight loss followed by rapid regain (as in bulimia) results in a net loss of lean body weight and a gain of fat weight.

PREVENTION AND TREATMENT OF EATING DISORDERS

Given all these negative effects of eating disorders, it is obvious that coaches should help prevent their athletes from developing them. Because we don't know exactly what causes eating disorders, it is difficult to draw up preventive strategies. But current research indicates that there are some things coaches can do. First, coaches should realize that they can strongly influence their athletes. Eating disorders can be triggered by a single offhand remark from someone the athlete considers very important. To comment on an individual's body size or to require weight loss without offering further guidance is to risk pushing a highly motivated, uninformed athlete into dangerous, unhealthy behaviors.

Identifying Realistic Weight Goals

Weight loss can be achieved safely only if the weight goal is realistic and based on body composition rather than weight-for-height standards. Use the skinfold appraisal techniques described in chapter 2. The athlete must eat sufficient calories to avoid the loss of muscle tissue, and he or she should start a weight loss program well before the season begins. The athlete should not lose more than 1 to 2 pounds per week. Monitor changes in body composition monthly with skinfold measures or hydrostatic weighing.

Provide Nutritional Guidance

Offer the athlete guidance and encouragement to practice safe weight loss techniques as outlined in chapter 11. A registered dietitian, if available, can help individuals plan low-fat, nutritionally adequate diets. Throughout this process, emphasize the importance of long-term good nutrition to performance and health, and don't overplay the value of low body weight.

Monitor Weight

After the athlete has reached the target weight, you should continue to monitor weight and body composition to detect any continued or unwarranted losses. The fat loss timetable described in chapter 11 allows you to see if the athlete is losing at an accelerated rate. Forbidding the athlete to practice or compete when weight loss becomes excessive is an effective tactic in preventing eating disorders.

Be Observant

Despite every effort to prevent them, eating disorders do occur. If you recognize symptoms of an eating disorder or are approached by concerned teammates and have reason to believe these concerns are valid, confront the athlete with the problem. Then meet with the athlete's parents to arrange for professional evaluation.

Seek Professional Help

Do not attempt to diagnose or treat anorexia nervosa or bulimia, but be specific about your suspicions and talk with the athlete about the fears or anxieties he or she may be having about performance or schoolwork. Help the athlete locate and contact an eating disorders clinic or professional screening center. If the athlete denies any problem but the evidence is to the contrary, consult a trained professional to decide on the next step.

Be a Team Member

The treatment of an athlete's eating disorder involves the joint efforts of a physician, a psychologist, a social worker, a nutritionist, and often the coach. After comprehensive evaluation, the members of the treatment team may meet separately with the athlete on a regular basis. Parents are involved to a greater or lesser extent, depending on the athlete's age and family circumstances. Hospitalization may eventually be required.

SUMMARY AND RECOMMENDATIONS

The prognosis for an athlete suffering from an eating disorder can be good. However, the mortality rate is from 5% to 15%; therefore the best approach is prevention. To help prevent your athletes from adopting behaviors that may lead to eating disorders, you should take the following steps:

1. Assume responsibility for providing your athletes with sound nutritional information. Administration of the Diet Habit Survey in Appendix B is a good way of telling your athletes about sound nutrition.

2. Emphasize energy management and performance enhancement rather than just weight loss.

3. Use the body composition techniques to emphasize fat loss rather than just weight loss.

4. Monitor your athletes' behavior as well as their weight loss. If you note abnormal weight patterns or any of the signs and symptoms of anorexia or bulimia that have been highlighted in this chapter, confront your athletes.

5. Seek out professionals in your community to whom you can refer athletes who may need evaluation and treatment for eating disorders.

Chapter 13
Eating to Gain Lean Weight

In chapter 11, we discussed how you can help your athletes lose excess fat weight to improve their physical efficiency. However, not all sports have the same performance demands, and thus their characteristics of physical efficiency vary. Some athletes, such as shot-putters, discus throwers, football linemen, and heavyweight wrestlers, require maximal muscle mass, needing both bulk and explosive strength. Remember, however, these athletes should increase their muscle weight, not just their body weight. Additional fat weight is just excess baggage; it does not contribute to the athlete's explosive strength potential. Furthermore, excess fat predisposes athletes, as they grow older, to a number of different diseases and other health problems.

Increases in muscle mass or lean body weight are of considerable importance to performance success in some sports. Therefore, the guidelines for gaining lean weight presented in this chapter are meant to supplement the fat loss guidelines discussed in chapter 11.

CALORIC BALANCE

Although gaining lean weight is considerably different than losing fat weight, the concept of caloric balance is the same. The emphasis, however, is on increased rather than reduced caloric intake. High caloric intake without an increase in body fat is possible only if intake is balanced by intense training, including resistive exercise. With this in mind let's look at the 10 guidelines for gaining lean weight.

Guidelines for Gaining Lean Weight

Check family medical histories

Increase caloric consumption

Eat a balanced diet

Eat a hearty breakfast

Eat frequently

Avoid animal fats and salty foods

Utilize heavy resistive training

Avoid using anabolic steroids

Be patient

Emphasize performance gains, not weight gains

Check Family Medical Histories

The athlete's age and the medical history of the athlete and his or her family should be considered before initiating any weight gain program. Although it is possible for prepubertal athletes to respond to strength training and weight gain programs, gains will be considerably greater for postpubertal athletes (Larsson, 1982). With younger athletes, the goals should not necessarily be weight gain but rather the development of sound dietary practices. Also, these prepubertal years should be an excellent time to master weight-lifting techniques before the emphasis is placed on overload for strength acquisition.

Athletes with a family history of heart disease or high blood pressure should see their family physicians before initiating a weight gain program. Blood pressure should be measured to determine whether to undertake or continue a weight gain program. If blood pressure is high initially, weight gain should be approached with caution and under the guidance of a physician. When possible, blood lipid profiles should be done to determine if abnormal levels of lipids, or fats, are present in the athlete's blood. Again, if these values are abnormally high be sure to involve a physician in any plans for weight gain.

Increase Caloric Consumption

Increased caloric consumption is essential for gaining lean tissue. Although the exact amount of the increase varies from athlete to athlete, Smith (1978) has suggested that a pound of lean tissue contains about 2,500 kilocalories (kcal). Fat, remember, contains about 3,500 kcal per pound. The difference in the number of kilocalories between these two tissues reflects the composition of the tissues. Lean tissue, such as muscle and nerve tissue, contains more protein, carbohydrate, and water than does adipose tissue. (Remember that one gram of fat contains about 9 kcal, and a gram of carbohydrate contains a little over 4 kcal. Water contains no kilocalories.)

Though most athletes recognize that they must eat more if they are to gain weight, coaches must guide this extra eating. Athletes should not engage in indiscriminate "pigging out." A great deal of science should go into structuring a weight gain program. Be sure to follow the guidelines and weight gain steps presented in this chapter as you structure weight gain programs for your athletes.

Eat a Balanced Diet

The increased calorie diet required for weight gain should be a *balanced* diet. A balanced diet, as you recall from chapter 11, is one in which 65% of the calories come from carbohydrates and only 20% come from fats. The high-carbohydrate foods provide lots of vitamins and minerals. Furthermore, with 15% of the calories coming from protein sources, adequate amino acids are available for muscle growth and other requirements. Under these conditions, as caloric intake increases, more amino acids (from proteins) are consumed, thus providing the body with the building blocks for tissue and enzyme synthesis.

Eat a Hearty Breakfast

The idea behind this guideline is to have your athletes consume the largest portion of their caloric intake early in the day. This helps to ensure that all requisite amino acids and other food components are eaten at about the same time, making it more likely that these substances will all be available to the body for tissue formation. Research has shown that all the constituents for building new tissues must be available simultaneously. The body is not able to hold what was eaten for breakfast until the rest of the ingredients are eaten for lunch. This is a major reason for eating balanced meals.

In addition to providing a supply of amino acids and other nutrients, eating a large portion of the caloric intake early in the day means that the food can be used for fuel during the active part of the day. A large meal eaten in the evening has a greater tendency to result in fat deposits than does a substantial breakfast. This is true not only for athletes but for everyone.

Eat Frequently

Although you'll want your athletes to eat a substantial breakfast and lunch, none of the meals that your athletes eat should be extremely large. Instead, players should eat extra "meals" throughout the day. Increased caloric consumption seems to be most easily achieved by adding snacks or mini-meals rather than eating one or two very large meals. Spreading out caloric consumption also helps to ensure optimal blood glucose levels and continued availability of amino acids for protein synthesis and recovery from workouts. As an added advantage, when the athlete no longer needs to gain weight, caloric intake can be reduced by cutting out snacks, still leaving the basic habit of consuming three balanced meals a day.

Avoid Animal Fats and Salty Foods

Research has demonstrated that a diet high in saturated fats (animal fats) may lead to an increased incidence of cardiovascular disease. In addition, a diet that has a high salt content may play a role in the development of hypertension, at least for some individuals. Therefore the increased caloric intake required for weight gain should come from foods that are low in saturated fats and salt.

You will need to provide specific instructions for your athletes because the traditional high-calorie foods that have been used in weight gain programs are high in saturated fat. For example, many young football players have learned to eat piles of scrambled eggs accompanied by slabs of bacon, and milk shakes made with whole milk, cream, and eggs to gain a few pounds. Granted, these types of foods increase caloric intake, but they also increase the athlete's fat intake. Consequently, such an athlete will no longer be consuming a balanced high-carbohydrate, low-fat diet.

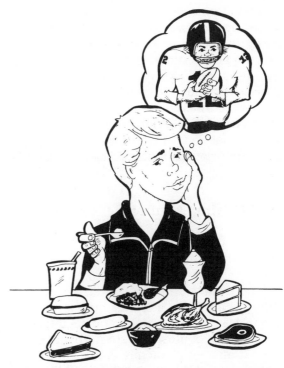

Figure 13.1. Gaining lean weight takes more than dreams and desserts; it takes intense resistive exercise.

Utilize Heavy Resistive Training

Increased caloric consumption should be coupled with heavy resistive exercise to gain lean weight or muscle weight (see Figure 13.1). In chapter 11, you learned that if caloric intake exceeds daily caloric output, the excess calories are stored as fat. However, if athletes not only increase their caloric intake but also work with weights and other training programs, their bodies will use the extra calories to build muscle tissue, other lean tissues, and the chemical enzymes necessary for muscle function.

By resistive exercise, we mean strength development exercises. Some excellent resources for developing these types of programs include the following:

Book	Authors	Publisher
Designing Resistance Training Programs	Fleck, S. & Kraemer, W.	Human Kinetics Champaign, IL
Weight Training for Everyone	Tuten, R., Moore, C., & Knight, V.	Hunter Publishing Winston-Salem, NC
Getting Stronger	Pearl, B.	Shelter Publications Bolinas, CA
Sports Conditioning and Weight Training	Stone, M. & Kroll, W.	Allyn and Bacon Boston, MA
Weight Training: A Scientific Approach	Stone, M. & O'Bryant, H.	Burgess Publishing Minneapolis, MN

Although the weight training programs discussed by these authorities result in increased strength, they can also be very stressful to growing bones. Very high-intensity strength training programs should not begin until after puberty when the growth of the long bones is near completion (American Academy of Pediatrics, 1983). Prior to this time, athletes can still use weight training but with higher numbers of repetitions and lighter weights.

Avoid Using Anabolic Steroids

Although the American College of Sports Medicine position statement (1984) on anabolic steroids stipulates that when taken in concert with high-calorie diets and intensive physical training, anabolic steroids probably do increase lean tissue weight and facilitate the development of muscular strength and endurance, it also emphatically states that taking anabolic steroids is dangerous and unhealthy. Anyone who takes anabolic steroids before he or she stops growing is likely to stunt growth because steroids can prematurely arrest the growth zones at the end of the long bones. Other side effects associated with anabolic steroids include acne, excessive body hair, enlargement of the breasts (because some of the steroid is converted to the female hormone estrogen), and deepening of the female voice. Due to these and other risk factors, as well as ethical considerations, the use of anabolic steroids has no place in the weight gain program of athletes—young or old! For a more complete review of the problem, the excellent position paper of the American College of Sports Medicine may be obtained by writing to the ACSM National Center, 401 W. Michigan Street, Indianapolis, IN 46202.

Be Patient

Lean weight gain will be slow and gradual even if you and your athletes adhere to all the information presented in the preceding guidelines. This is because the extra calories that are being consumed must be taken into cells and used to synthesize new lean tissues and the associated enzymes for energy release. These processes take time, especially in the

teenage athlete who is undergoing rapid growth.

If too many calories are consumed in too short a time, a disproportionate amount of the weight gain will be fat weight. The exact daily increase is not known, but generally speaking, the athlete's weight gain should be limited to 0.5 to 1 pound per week. The gain of 0.5 pounds per week is probably most realistic for the small athlete (100 to 150 pounds) and the 1-pound-per-week goal is probably reasonable for the larger athlete (150 to 200 pounds). If, as was stated earlier, a pound of lean tissue contains 2,500 kilocalories, a *minimum* of 1,250 extra kilocalories must be consumed each week for an increase of 0.5 pounds of lean weight. The word minimum was used because some athletes have to eat more to achieve the same gain in lean tissue. It is critical that coaches not have unrealistic weight gain expectations for their athletes.

Emphasize Performance Gains, Not Weight Gains

It takes time for lean weight gains to occur; however, if athletes are involved in good training programs, their strength, power, quickness, and other performance attributes will improve. By tracking these improvements and monitoring skinfold thickness, coaches can reinforce the concept that performance improvement, not just weight gain, is the real goal. Even if the weight gain is not up to the athlete's ultimate weight goal, improvements in strength and conditioning translate into better performances on the field, in the gym, or on the court.

STEPS TO IMPLEMENTING A WEIGHT GAIN PROGRAM

Now that you know the guidelines, let's take a look at the steps for implementing a weight gain program.

Weight Gain Steps

Step 1: Determine if weight gain is necessary

Step 2: Consider the impact of weight gain on the athlete's health

Step 3: Evaluate the athlete's dietary habits

Step 4: Establish specific dietary goals

Step 5: Initiate a resistive exercise program

Step 6: Monitor weight gain

Step 7: Reevaluate your athletes

Determine If Weight Gain Is Necessary

Determine the athlete's body composition and decide on the gain in muscle tissue necessary. You may use the skinfold procedures presented in chapter 2 to estimate percent fat and fat-free weight, but use your common sense to establish reasonable weight gain goals. For example, if a football player has a lower body weight than other players but a percent fat and stature similar to those who play at the same position, the athlete's goal should be to gain lean tissue.

Consider the Impact of Weight Gain on the Athlete's Health

As mentioned previously, athletes who have high blood pressure or a family history of hypertension or other cardiovascular diseases should seek input from their physicians before undertaking a weight gain program. Study the information from the athlete's preparticipation physical examination. More specifically, ask these questions:

- Is the athlete's blood pressure above 140/90?
- Does the athlete's family have a history of hypertension or high blood pressure?

You should also note the athlete's age. Prepubertal athletes do not have the hormones to significantly increase body size, and an athlete in the midst of a growth spurt will find it difficult to achieve additional increases in muscle mass.

Evaluate the Athlete's Dietary Habits

Once you and the athlete have determined that lean weight gain is necessary and appar-ently not harmful, evaluate the athlete's present nutritional habits and practices by having him or her complete the Diet Habit Survey (Connor & Connor, 1986) that was introduced in chapter 11. (A copy of this survey is found in Appendix B.) Although this step requires some time, it is time well spent. In completing the survey the athlete is taking an active role in determining his or her own destiny. The survey score provides a tool for evaluating the athlete's eating habits. If these habits are less than optimal, which is typical for most Americans, the survey also serves as a guide for identifying nutritional goals for the athlete.

Establish Specific Dietary Goals

The goal for optimal nutrition for the athlete involved in a weight gain program is for the athlete to score above the Phase III point total on all the survey categories. This can probably best be accomplished by eating a good breakfast, lunch, and dinner and by adding one to three high-carbohydrate, high-protein, low-fat snacks to the diet. Some ideas for these snacks are presented here.

High-Calorie-Density Snacks

Nuts:
  Cashews
  Peanuts
  Almonds
  Walnuts

Coconut

Milk

Chocolate milk

Sherbet (provides the same sugar calories as ice cream without the animal fat)

Sherbet sundaes with nuts, wheat germ, and coconut topping

Milk shakes and malts

Cheese

Dried fruit (without its water content, fruit is very high in calories)

Peanut butter sandwiches

Initially, these snacks should add 300 to 500 kilocalories to the athlete's daily caloric intake. Emphasis was placed on high-bulk foods such as fresh fruit, salads, and high-fiber cereals when fat loss was the primary goal. These types of foods, however, are too filling to constitute a very high percentage of the dietary intake necessary for weight gain. Rather, the athlete must eat high-calorie-density foods to gain lean weight. Dried fruit, for example, has a much higher calorie density than fresh fruit; consequently, dried fruits are an excellent snack food for the weight gain eating plan.

Low-fat protein snacks are also appropriate, but it is not necessary for athletes to stuff themselves with large quantities of expensive meat to bulk up on protein. Although athletes trying to gain weight do need somewhat more protein than their sedentary counterparts, the quantity of protein required can easily be met if 15% to 20% of the total calories consumed are protein. This type of a balanced diet easily provides the 2 to 2.5 grams of protein per kilogram of body weight (slightly more than a gram per pound) necessary for optimal gains in fat-free weight. Chicken, turkey, the white of a hard-boiled egg, water-packed tuna, and skim milk are excellent sources of low-fat protein.

There are also numerous protein tablets or supplements on the market. They are not necessary if the athlete takes care to eat natural high-quality protein foods throughout the day. If protein supplements are used, however, Crooks (1975) recommends that they be developed from animal sources. Remember, too, that it is not necessary to consume more than 2 to 2.5 grams per kilogram of body weight. For a 150-pound (or 68-kilogram) athlete, this means 136 to 170 grams of protein. This could easily be achieved with a diet similar to that portrayed in Table 13.1. You should, however, discuss high-calorie meal plans with your athletes and their parents.

Initiate a Resistive Exercise Program

If your athletes are not already in a weight training program, you need to begin one. (Recommended readings on this subject were given on page 121.) Remember that it takes considerable time for athletes to work up to being able to engage in heavy resistive training, so be patient with your athletes.

Once the desired weight gain has been achieved, the athlete should stop excessive caloric consumption and begin a maintenance weight training program. In addition, if the caloric expenditure is reduced when the season ends or if the athlete incurs an injury, caloric intake should be reduced. High caloric intake without an increase in body fat is possible only when balanced by intensive training programs.

Monitor Weight Gain

Establish a procedure for monitoring the weight gain process. The weight loss timetable presented in chapter 11 could be modified and used as a tool for tracking gains in fat-free weight. You can also use girth measurements, skinfold measurements, sprint times, strength scores, and other performance indices to evaluate the efficacy of the weight gain. Figure 13.2 (see page 126) illustrates one way you can record the necessary information. With the measurements available you can evaluate the success of the program. If, for example, weight and fat-free weight go up, skinfold thicknesses also go up, and performance deteriorates, you can conclude that the athlete has not benefited from the weight gain.

If after several weeks of increased caloric intake and heavy training you do not see some increase in fat-free weight, further adjustments are necessary. The following step provides some guidance for these adjustments.

Reevaluate Your Athletes

In the previous steps we suggested that a considerable amount of information be collected on each athlete, including body composition, body weight, performance scores, and dietary information. Although there is some value in a single collection of such information, the real value is in looking at changes in this information that occur over time. Skinfold thickness and changes in body weight can be used to evaluate the impact of the weight gain program on body composition. Changes in performance scores tell you whether the program is enhancing performance, and information about dietary habits helps you see if the athlete is making progress in changing eating habits.

Table 13.1

A Sample High-Calorie Diet for Gaining Muscle Weight (6,027 kcal)

Breakfast	Lunch	Dinner	Snacks
1 glass skim milk (90 kcal)	1 glass skim milk (90 kcal)	Large baked potato with sour cream and margarine (280 kcal)	1 c dried peaches and other dried fruits (420 kcal)
1 glass cranberry juice cocktail (165 kcal)	1 chicken breast—6 oz (310 kcal)	6 oz baked fish (300 kcal)	1 pt sherbet (400 kcal)
1 soft-boiled egg (80 kcal)	1 c rice with cheese sauce (315 kcal)	1 c creamed broccoli casserole with sesame seeds on top (350 kcal)	1 glass orange juice (80 kcal)
2 pieces whole-wheat toast (130 kcal)	Tossed salad with dressing (200 kcal)	½ c cottage cheese with pears (200 kcal)	½ c peanuts (392 kcal)
1½ t margarine (105 kcal)	1 c fruit cocktail (190 kcal)	2 dinner rolls with margarine (310 kcal)	1 milk shake (320 kcal)
1 T jelly (50 kcal)	4 oatmeal-and-raisin cookies (240 kcal)	1 piece of apple pie (400 kcal)	½ c gorp (granola, dried fruits, chocolate bits, nuts, and coconut [250 kcal])
½ c granola (260 kcal)			1 banana (100 kcal)

Criteria for Evaluating Weight Gain

Purpose of the weight gain program _____

_____

Weight gain goal _____ Target time _____

Criteria	Date	Date	Date	Date	Date	Date
1. Body weight						
2. Subscapular skinfold						
3. Triceps skinfold						
4. 20 yd sprint time						
5. 50 yd sprint time						
6. Waist girth						
7. Upper-arm girth						
8. Calf girth						
9. Chest girth						
10. Bench press						
11. Other						

Figure 13.2.   You can monitor weight gain by using forms similar to this one.

Although athletes don't need to keep track of their caloric consumption on a daily basis, they should always be aware of what types of foods to avoid, the types of foods to select, the way to balance hard work and rest, and the importance of regular sleep and eating patterns to optimal weight gain. To help your athletes with this information have them retake the Diet Habit Survey every 3 to 4 weeks during the season. A simple daily log, such as the one shown here, can also be used to monitor training and sleep patterns.

Training Log

Athlete's name: _____   Date: _____

Total number of pounds lifted: _____   Total number of reps.: _____

Went to bed at:_____   Got up at: _____

Nap minutes:_____   Total hours of sleep:_____

Quality of sleep: _____

Overall daily stress rating:
_____

High   Medium high   Average   Medium low   Low

Comments:

If your athlete is getting closer to Phase III on the Diet Habit Survey, is training hard, and is sleeping a sufficient number of hours regularly and fat-free weight is still not increasing, the quantity (number and size of portions) of extra food items may need to be increased. Even if your athletes are gaining weight, re-evaluation is still important. The information you collect allows you to see if the weight gain is resulting in improved performance.

SUMMARY AND RECOMMENDATIONS

For some sports and activities, physical size is a valuable attribute. Several factors can influence the development of physical size—probably the most important is the athlete's genetic potential. Some athletes gain lean weight more easily and thus enhance their performance potential in certain sports more than other athletes. Remember this fact and communicate it to your athletes, but also emphasize to them that they all can benefit from training hard and adopting good dietary habits. Show your athletes how to facilitate hard training by adopting a scientific approach to their eating habits. To accomplish this you should take the following steps:

1. Use the calipers technique to calculate the body composition of your athletes. This information, as well as body weight and size, will enable you to determine if a given athlete should gain lean weight.
2. Determine if weight gain will be hazardous to the athlete's long-term health.
3. Incorporate resistive exercise into your athletes' training programs.
4. Administer the Diet Habit Survey to your athletes and use it to set eating goals.
5. Instruct your athletes to eat a balanced diet consisting of three meals and two or three high-carbohydrate, high-protein snacks.
6. Establish a procedure for monitoring the weight gain process by tracking such variables as fat-free weight, skinfold thickness, girth measurements, and performance indices.
7. Reevaluate the dietary and lifestyle habits of your athletes by using the Diet Habit Survey and the daily training log presented. Evaluate the results of these tools every 3 or 4 weeks during the season.
8. Demonstrate your realization that not all athletes will gain lean weight at the same rate by being patient with your athlete's weight gain progress.
9. Remember that performance enhancement, not just weight gain for its own sake, is the ultimate goal.

Chapter 14
The High-Performance Eating Plan

A high-performance eating plan is one that provides adequate quantities of vitamins, minerals, water, and protein as well as optimal quantities of the high-energy fuel foods. It is an eating plan designed to optimize performance by making energy fuels available to the muscles and nerves. The purpose of this chapter is not to suggest that specific foods are a substitute for training, practice, and body fat control, but to emphasize that the content of the food eaten during prolonged exercise bouts and between hard training sessions can influence the quality of training. In addition, the meals that an athlete eats in the days prior to competition can influence athletic performance.

MUSCLE GLYCOGEN

The concept behind a high-performance diet is the culmination of much research. This research has demonstrated that dietary carbohydrates or starches are broken down in digestion into simple sugars and that these simple sugars (primarily glucose) are taken up by the muscle and liver cells and stored as glycogen. Still other research has shown that although fat is the major fuel for low- to moderate-intensity exercise, as exercise intensity increases the body depends more and more on glucose from stored muscle as well as on liver glycogen for energy (see chapter 5).

Some researchers speculate that the amount of muscle glycogen an athlete has limits his or her endurance capacities. A series of studies by Swedish physiologists verified this con-

cept (Bergstrom & Hultman, 1972; Hultman & Bergstrom, 1967). In these studies, the amount of glycogen in the muscle was sampled before and after endurance exercise. The researchers observed that the greater the initial stores of muscle glycogen, the longer the activity could be sustained and that the time to exhaustion was closely related to the emptying of these stores (see Figure 14.1). Therefore, coaches of athletes in high-intensity, strenuous sports such as wrestling and gymnastics as well as coaches of athletes in endurance sports like distance running should be particularly concerned with having their athletes optimize muscle glycogen storage.

OPTIMIZING MUSCLE GLYCOGEN

If the goal is to optimize muscle glycogen storage, an obvious question is raised: Can the amount of glycogen stored in the muscle be altered or enhanced by manipulating the diet? Over the years, in attempts to answer this question, athletes have been fed many different types of food. In one study (Bergstrom, Hermansen, Hultman, & Saltin, 1967), a normal diet, a diet limited to protein and fat, and a high-carbohydrate diet were compared (see Figure 14.2). While the subjects were on the normal diet, muscle glycogen concentrations averaged 1.75 grams per 100 grams of muscle. After 3 days of a high-protein, high-fat diet with low carbohydrate intake, muscle glycogen levels fell to 0.6 grams per 100 grams of muscle. However, when much of the fat in the

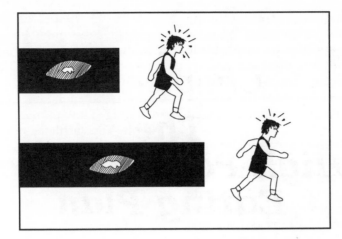

Figure 14.1.   The larger the quantity of stored glycogen in the muscle, the longer physical activity can be sustained.

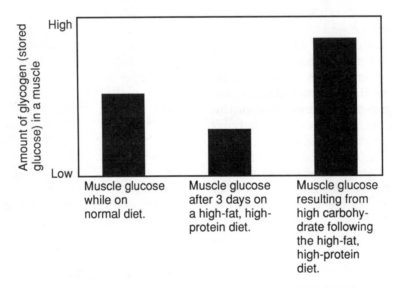

Figure 14.2.   The amount of glucose stored in the muscles can be altered by diet.

menu was replaced with carbohydrate, subjects stored twice as much muscle glycogen as they had on the normal diet (3.4 grams per 100 grams of muscle). So it seems that diet can influence the amount of glycogen stored.

CARBOHYDRATE LOADING

Findings such as these led to the development of a dietary strategy for athletes known as *carbohydrate loading*. When done properly, carbohydrate loading results in muscle glycogen levels two to three times above normal. However, this technique is not without its drawbacks and is certainly not appropriate for

every sport. Although carbohydrate loading has been replaced by other less risky methods for optimizing glycogen stores, it is of interest to many coaches, and so we will describe it.

Depletion Phase

If you are going to have your athletes use this technique, you need to schedule a training session 6 days before competition that results in the depletion of the athlete's muscle glycogen stores. Such a session should be 70 to 90 minutes in duration and fairly intense (at about 70% of maximal effort). The exercises or activities that you select for this session must utilize the same muscle groups that the athlete will use for the competition, because glycogen stores are specific to the muscle groups. In other words, a distance runner needs to deplete his or her stores by running. You also need to remember that the greater the depletion, the greater the final glycogen stores will be.

To prevent replenishment of the glycogen stores, have your athletes consume a high-protein, high-fat diet for the next 3 days. They should eat a small amount of carbohydrate (100 grams or 400 kilocalories per day) during this period so that the brain and the rest of the nervous system have a supply of glucose for fuel.

Loading Phase

During the 3 days prior to the competition, have your athletes switch to a high-carbohydrate diet. During the loading phase, carbohydrates should provide at least 75% of the total calories. Total caloric consumption, however, should not exceed the maintenance level for your athletes. The idea is for your athletes to "overfill" the glycogen reserves of their muscles, not to gorge themselves so much that they gain fat weight.

During this period, you should also taper down or cut back on your athletes' training and practice schedule. After being starved for glycogen, the athletes' muscles overcompensate and store two to three times the usual amount of glycogen. The reduced training load ensures that the newly stored muscle glycogen is not used until the day of competition.

Hazards

There are several drawbacks to this classical carbohydrate loading technique. Let's examine the most important of these.

Too Much Fat

During the first 3 days of the carbohydrate loading plan, athletes consume an excessive amount of fat, which can cause indigestion and nausea. In addition, your athletes may feel weak and irritable during the depletion phase

due to the lack of carbohydrate in the diet and the subsequent rise of acids in the blood (known as ketones) resulting from the fat breakdown. The depletion phase also affects training. Because the glycogen stores become lower with each successive day of depletion, training at an optimal level becomes more difficult. Your athletes may feel stale, as if they have no speed or power in their legs. Training through such fatigue may place athletes at a higher risk of injury.

Weight Gain

During the loading phase, when your athletes suddenly reintroduce large amounts of carbohydrate into their diet, their muscles store the glucose as glycogen. Because three parts of water are stored for each part of glycogen, your athletes can easily gain 3 to 5 pounds. Such weight gain may cause them feelings of sluggishness or muscle stiffness and may adversely affect performance in activities where the body's weight is lifted, or where agility is required. In addition, the sudden change to a high-carbohydrate diet may cause your athletes to suffer intestinal distress and nausea. More serious are the irregular heartbeats and cardiac abnormalities that have been observed among some athletes who have engaged in carbohydrate loading.

Time Limitations

If the carbohydrate loading technique is used more than two or three times a year, less glycogen is stored each time. Because most sports require competitions more frequently than once a year, some different approaches to optimizing muscle glycogen are indicated. In addition, only activities that last well over an hour benefit from carbohydrate loading.

No Fuel for Training

Perhaps the greatest limitation of the classical carbohydrate loading strategy is that it does not provide for your athletes' day-to-day energy needs. As we stated earlier, a special diet before competition cannot compensate for poor training. Quality training makes for better athletes, and a major determinant of quality training is the ability of the athlete to *work hard* during practice and training sessions.

Your athletes will not be able to work hard if they do not replace their muscle glycogen levels on a daily basis. An interesting study by Costill, Bowers, Branam, & Sparks (1971) demonstrated that this daily muscle glycogen replacement is not possible if athletes eat a low-carbohydrate diet. (In the typical American diet only 45% of kilocalories come from carbohydrate.) Muscle glycogen levels are maintained only if diets contain 70% carbohydrate. Coaches should also note that when the athletes in this study were on the low-carbohydrate diet, they felt that the training was very hard; when they were on the high-carbohydrate diet, they did not feel that way.

Because of these potential problems and because sport scientists have documented that adequate muscle glycogen levels can be achieved without the high-fat, high-protein portion of the depleting phase, we suggest that you *not* have your athletes utilize the classic carbohydrate loading plan. Instead, we believe that the research literature supports the high-performance eating plan presented in the following section. You will notice that this plan still calls for a high-carbohydrate diet, but there is no dramatic switching back and forth between this diet and a high-fat, high-protein one.

EATING FOR HIGH PERFORMANCE

The goal of the high-performance eating plan is to work toward a diet that is about 65% carbohydrate (Phase III on the Diet Habit Survey) and to help your athletes translate this goal into real food. Simply adding carbohydrates to the typical American diet probably will not produce optimal results, because the typical diet includes too much fat. In fact, most Americans get approximately 40% of their total kilocalories from fats.

One reason that most Americans eat too much fat is because they use fats and oils to prepare most foods. Foods that are naturally low in fat on the cupboard shelf become high-fat foods on the plate. For example, many coaches believe that a spaghetti dinner provides their athletes with a high-carbohydrate meal. Most people, however, do not eat their pasta plain but instead smother it in a rich sauce made with lots of oil, then add a few

slices of garlic bread soaked in butter and a large piece of Italian sausage served on the side. In this way a potentially high-carbohydrate meal actually becomes a high-fat meal instead.

Although many Americans are reducing their meat intake in an effort to lower their total intake of saturated (animal) fat, there is evidence that reducing total fats, both saturated and unsaturated, is at least as important as reducing saturated fat. Therefore, our ideal high-performance eating plan calls for reduction of fat intake regardless of the source—animal or vegetable.

Reduce Fat Intake

For athletes, the need to reduce fat is even greater than for nonathletes, because they need to replenish muscle glycogen between daily workouts and practice sessions. Only dietary carbohydrates can be used to replace muscle glycogen; dietary fat cannot be converted to carbohydrates in the body. Consequently, coaches need to encourage their athletes to eat substantial quantities of carbohydrates. However, if athletes accomplish this by eating more carbohydrates that are prepared with fats, the result is a high-calorie diet. Such a diet leads to increased fat storage. Increased fat storage means increased fat weight and, for any sport that requires moving the body against gravity, that translates into a decrease in performance.

Increase Carbohydrate Intake

The trick to a successful high-carbohydrate diet is to help your athletes and their parents understand that whenever possible they must eliminate fat from the diet and replace it with high-carbohydrate substitutes. For example, many high-fat foods, such as sauces, salad dressings, cheeses, meats, and ice cream, are available in low-fat (usually called diet) forms.

Low-fat versions of popular foods mentioned above have reduced kilocalories when compared with the originals, but more importantly, the kilocalories have been reduced by replacing fat normally used as thickeners with natural carbohydrate-based stabilizers. Admittedly, the names of these stabilizers—guar gum, gum carrageenan, xanthine gum—sound somewhat ominous. They are, however, naturally occurring carbohydrates that are lower in kilocalories and probably safer to eat than the fats they replace. Table 14.1 includes some high-carbohydrate, low-fat replacements for common foods.

Table 14.1
Recommended Replacements
to Increase Carbohydrate Intake
and Decrease Fat Intake

Food item	Replace with
Bologna	Turkey ham
Cheese	Reduced-calorie dressing
Mayonnaise	Mustard
Red meat	Chicken, fish
Salad dressing	Reduced-calorie dressing
Sour cream	Plain yogurt
Oil-packed tuna	Water-packed tuna
High-fat cookies	Gingersnaps, Fig Newtons

Many of the low-fat substitutes require that your athletes cultivate some new tastes. This process of changing the diet can often be made easier by doing it gradually, in phases. The three choice phases presented in Table 14.2 offer a strategy for gradually introducing change into the athlete's diet. The selection phases correspond to the Diet Habit Survey assessment forms.

Coaches should also share the following suggestions with athletes and their parents:

- Use Pam or similar spray-type, vegetable-based products to coat pans for cooking.
- Reduce the number of egg yolks in omelets and scrambled eggs.
- Examine labels and observe where fat is listed. The farther down the list, the better.
- Avoid high-fat cookies and pastries.

The Right Amount of Carbohydrate

Although it is easy to say that the goal is for athletes to consume 65% to 70% of their calories as carbohydrates, calculation of exactly what that means is a bit more difficult. There are, however, a couple of approaches to this task. One is to use the Diet Habit Survey introduced in chapter 11. If you have your athletes complete this survey, their total scores can be used to specify how much carbohydrate they need to consume to achieve the goal of 65% carbohydrate intake. For the athlete to reach this goal, he or she must score at the Phase III level on the survey.

Another approach to determine how much carbohydrate translates into 65% of the calories is to multiply the athlete's weight in kilograms by 5. This gives you the number of grams of carbohydrate that the athlete should consume on a daily basis. Before you can complete this multiplication process, you must first calculate your athlete's weight in kilograms (kg). This is done by dividing the athlete's weight in pounds (lb) by 2.2. For example, if Jay weighs 132 lb, his weight is

Table 14.2
Gradual Modification of the Diet Through Choice Phases

Standard choice	Good choice	Better choice	Best choice
Butter	Margarine	Light spread	Diet margarine
Whole milk cottage cheese	2% butterfat cottage cheese	1% butterfat cottage cheese	0.5% butterfat cottage cheese
Ice cream	Frozen yogurt	Ice milk	Fruit sorbet
Mayonnaise	Light mayonnaise	Diet mayonnaise	Mustard
Whole milk	2% milk	1% milk	Skim/nonfat milk
Yogurt	Low-fat yogurt	—	Non-fat yogurt

60 kg (132 lb/2.2 = 60 kg). Now, if you multiply 60 kg by 5 you will calculate that Jay needs to consume 300 grams of carbohydrate daily (60 kg × 5 grams per kg = 300).

The information in Appendix C can now be used to select the appropriate amount of carbohydrate. For example, Jay can fulfill his need for 250 grams of carbohydrate by eating the following foods:

Food selection	Grams of carbohydrate
Bowl of cereal	35
3 bananas	57
1 apple	22
4 slices of bread	56
Baked potato	33
2-3 Fig Newtons	33
Mixed vegetables	24
Chocolate ice milk	54

Total carbohydrates = 314 grams

Of course these carbohydrates need to be consumed along with protein sources and some fat. An example of how this can be accomplished may be seen in the low-fat meal plans presented in Table 14.3. We recommend replacement of granola-type cereals, which are actually high in fat, with regular flaked cereal. Similarly, replace whole milk with 2%, 1%, or skim milk, and replace yogurt made from whole milk with yogurt made from nonfat milk. For lunch, we have replaced the high-fat bologna with a lower-fat turkey ham product. High-fat cheese has been replaced with a low-fat "diet" cheese, and mayonnaise has been replaced with mustard. The advantage of wheat bread over white bread is primarily its higher fiber content. Instead of high-fat chocolate chip cookies, we used lower-fat Fig Newtons. Finally, we replaced the Almond Joy bar and corn chips with an apple and two bananas.

For dinner, we recommend lower-fat meats such as poultry (without the skin) and fish instead of higher-fat cuts of meat such as hamburger. Sour cream is lower in fat than butter and therefore a better choice. An excellent low-fat sour cream dressing can be made by mixing equal quantities of sour cream and nonfat yogurt. Substituting a low-fat dressing on the dinner salad is highly recommended. Finally, notice the addition of two slices of bread on the low-fat diet column. For dessert, avoid high-fat premium products and replace them with lower-fat equivalents. In Table 14.3 we have replaced ice cream with ice milk.

The low-fat diet provides 352 grams of carbohydrate versus 315 for the typical American diet. Perhaps even more important is the fact that this is accomplished with 1,200 fewer total calories. Following the low-fat diet, an athlete can easily meet increased carbohydrate requirements simply by increasing the total food intake. With the typical American diet, however, increasing total food intake to provide more carbohydrates may raise the level of total calories to the point that caloric balance is disturbed, resulting in unwanted fat gain.

The Best Carbohydrate Sources

The best carbohydrates to consume on the high-performance eating plan are complex carbohydrates. Complex carbohydrates such as whole-grain cereals, breads, rice, pasta, potatoes, fruits, and vegetables offer the most nutrition for the amount of calories they contain. Some simple carbohydrates, such as sugar, honey, candy, cookies, and sweetened drinks, are sources of energy, but they are usually low in vitamins and other nutrients. For this reason, the high-performance eating plan doesn't emphasize these simple sugars. However, during multiple-day competitions or tournaments, sports drinks and other simple sugar sources may be useful. The use of these products is discussed in more detail later in this chapter.

SPORT-SPECIFIC EATING PLANS

Although it is generally true that athletes need to consume a high-carbohydrate diet, there are some subtle differences between the requirements of endurance sports and those of power sports. Let's examine these differences.

Endurance Sports

The endurance athlete uses glycogen very efficiently over a long period of time. Therefore, large glycogen stores are essential. For

THE PRE-EVENT MEAL

Sports in general are frequently steeped in mythology and superstition. Socks are not washed once a winning streak begins, certain shirts are considered lucky, and many pregame or precompetition procedures have become rituals. Unfortunately, some of these rituals violate what sport scientists have learned. The traditional pregame meal of steak and eggs is just such a ritual that does not make sense from a scientific standpoint. Remember, protein and fat, which are the primary constituents of a steak-and-egg meal, are *not* the primary fuel the athlete needs— carbohydrates are. That is why the high-performance eating plan is dependent upon a diet high in carbohydrates.

Carbohydrates are also the key ingredient for the optimal pre-event or precompetition meal. Even though optimal muscle glycogen stores are the result of foods eaten days, not hours, before competition, the precompetition meal is important because it does contribute to liver glycogen levels. It is the liver that releases its glycogen as glucose so that blood glucose levels are maintained throughout the competition. The brain and nerves depend on blood glucose for their fuel supply. Consequently, the precompetition meal deserves attention.

Hunger Prevention

The first consideration for the precompetition meal is that the meal's caloric content should be sufficient to prevent feelings of hunger or weakness prior to and during the competitive event. A meal containing 500 kilocalories can easily serve to maintain the athlete's blood sugar at a level that ensures adequate fuel for the brain and nerves.

Quick Digestion

The most easily digested, absorbed, and ready source of blood sugar is carbohydrate. Carbohydrates leave the stomach more quickly than either protein or fat and should provide the majority of the pre-event meal calories. Sample 500-kilocalorie pre-event meals are shown in Table 14.4. Avoid high-fiber foods, spicy ingredients, foods high in fat, and any food that is unfamiliar. Ideally, the pre-event

Table 14.4
Sample Pre-Event Meals

Morning competition

2 corn muffins, 1 t jam, 1 c skim milk, ½ grapefruit

1 whole English muffin, 1 t jelly, 1 c nonfat fruit yogurt, ½ c orange juice

1 c cream of wheat, 1 c skim milk, 1 t sugar, 1 c grapefruit juice

Afternoon or evening competition

Turkey or chicken sandwich on white bread with 1 t mustard, ½ banana, 1 c orange juice

6 saltines, ½ c 0.5% butterfat cottage cheese, ½ c fruit cocktail, ½ c apple juice

1 c pasta with tomato sauce, 1 slice French bread, ½ c skim milk, ½ c applesauce

meal should be eaten 3 to 4 hours before competition to allow the stomach to empty completely. Some athletes are particularly nervous before competition, which can slow stomach emptying time even further and cause gastrointestinal distress.

If gastric discomfort is a problem, a liquid pre-event meal might be the solution. Liquid meals empty from the stomach quickly and are low in residue. Several commercial liquid meals are available, and several brands are listed on page 138. These meals are high in carbohydrate polymers and contain sufficient protein and fat to give athletes a satisfied feeling and relieve hunger.

If your athletes are not familiar with liquid meals, have them experiment with them prior to actually using them on the day of competition. It is important that these products be prepared according to the directions and not doctored up or made too concentrated. Carbohydrate or glucose polymer solutions and supplements are less concentrated and cause less gastrointestinal distress than those high in sucrose, glucose, or other simple sugars. In addition, glucose polymers are absorbed at a more even rate than sugars, resulting in a more gradual and controlled rise in blood sugar levels.

Carbohydrate High

In some athletes, if blood sugar rises too rapidly they experience a period of feeling good followed by a drastic reduction in energy. The

Commercial Liquid Meals

Trade name	Manufacturer
Compete	Ross Laboratories
Exceed	Ross Laboratories
Osmolite	Ross Laboratories .
Isocal	Mead Johnson
Isosource	Sandoz
Sugar-Free Instant Breakfast	Carnation

period of feeling good is sometimes called a *carbohydrate high.* The "down" feeling that sometimes follows the "high" is due to a rapid drop in blood glucose. In these individuals, a rapid rise in blood glucose after drinking or eating glucose causes the body to secrete too much insulin—the hormone that lowers blood sugar levels. The result is low blood sugar and fatigue at a time when the athlete needs to be energetic.

As an example, a gymnastic coach decided to have a break during a 5-hour practice. He had the gymnasts bring fruit juice. They drank it, felt good for a while, but then had a hard time maintaining the intensity required for a quality practice. At the next 5-hour practice, the coach tried having the gymnasts drink cold water and eat a piece of fruit during their break. Presto! The second half of practice was excellent. Whole fruit, such as a banana or grapes, is high-carbohydrate food, but its energy is released more slowly than the energy in juice. Substituting a complex carbohydrate (fruit) for a simpler carbohydrate (juice) prevented the gymnasts from oversecreting insulin and "bottoming out."

FUEL REPLACEMENT DURING ACTIVITY

In chapter 9 we emphasized that your athletes need to replace the water they lose during exercise. This can be accomplished by drinking either water or sport drinks. If your athletes are exercising for 2 hours or longer, replacement of the fuel used during the event is as im-portant as or more important than eating carbohydrate foods the week before. Blood glucose may have dropped, and performance begins to fail if carbohydrates aren't provided during activity. This is true whether the activity is continuous or intermittent, as during a tournament or meet situation.

The easiest way to provide carbohydrates and to satisfy thirst is to make use of one of the sport drinks now available. The carbohydrates in sport drinks can be either simple sugars (fructose, sucrose, glucose) or complex sugars (glucose polymers). Some researchers contend that glucose polymers are more readily emptied from the stomach and absorbed into the body than simple sugars. Many athletes prefer these drinks because they don't have the undesirable too-sweet taste or stomach-upsetting properties of simple sugars at high concentrations.

Until recently, many sport scientists recommended that a sport drink contain no more than 2.5% carbohydrate. There is emerging evidence, however, that 2.5% is too conservative. In a study performed at the University of Texas (Coyle, Coggan, Hemmert, & Ivy, 1986), trained cyclists rode bicycles at 70% of their maximal aerobic power until they were fatigued. They were given either a placebo (artificially sweetened water) or a glucose polymer solution. The latter was taken at 50% concentration at the 20th minute of exercise, and at 10% concentration thereafter. When subjects were given placebos, they fatigued at 3 hours. When they were given glucose polymer solutions, they could exercise one hour longer.

Deciding which product to use is a choice that you should have your athletes make well before the day of competition. You and your athletes need to experiment with different types of solutions during practice and training sessions. Criteria for choosing products include the following:

- *Taste.* A pleasant flavor should hold up over time and in hot weather.
- *Concentration.* Although recommendations vary, the ideal percentage of carbohydrate for a sport drink seems to be from 2.5% to 10%. Anything higher may impede stomach emptying. See which works best for your athletes.
- *Electrolytes.* Athletes rarely become deficient in electrolytes during activity so the electrolyte concentration of the sport drink does not have to be too high.

After the choice of drink has been made, it is important to drink enough during the activity. A rule of thumb is to drink 5 to 8 ounces every 20 minutes. At this rate, a 10% carbohydrate drink replaces about 260 kilocalories per hour, helps maintain blood sugar levels, and possibly spares the use of muscle glycogen for fuel. If some of your athletes are trying to lose fat weight, they should be very cautious about consuming sport drinks. An athlete can easily drink several hundred kilocalories.

Also keep in mind the material on water toxicity that was presented in chapter 9. An athlete needs to replace only the fluids that are lost. If the exercise intensity is low and little sweat loss occurs, there is no need to drink 5 to 8 ounces every 20 minutes. In fact, such a practice could be dangerous.

SUMMARY AND RECOMMENDATIONS

Throughout this book we have praised the virtues of carbohydrates as the premier fuel for the athlete. In this chapter we have outlined a plan for optimizing carbohydrate consumption. Now that you have read this information, you should be ready to implement the high-performance eating plan in your program. To do this you must take the following steps:

1. Convince your athletes and their parents of the merits of a high-carbohydrate diet.
2. Help your athletes recognize that a high-carbohydrate diet can be achieved only if the diet is also low in fat.
3. Inform your athletes about which foods are high in carbohydrates. If you have your athletes take the Diet Habit Survey, they can see what types of food selections will increase the percent of carbohydrate in their diets. Appendix C also contains numerous examples of high-carbohydrate foods.
4. Encourage your athletes to start making dietary choices that decrease the fat content and increase the carbohydrate content of their diets.
5. Set 65% to 70% carbohydrate intake as the goal for endurance athletes and 65% as the goal for power athletes.
6. Encourage your athletes to eat high-carbohydrate meals 4 to 5 hours before competition. Have the athletes try these meals before practices to see if they tolerate the foods well.
7. Experiment with sport drinks during practice sessions in preparation for tournaments and meets that require multiple competitions. Be careful that athletes who are trying to lose fat weight do not consume large quantities of sport drinks. Remember, the purpose is to replace fuel that has been used.

The meals and snacks that athletes eat in the days immediately prior to competition can influence their performance. Athletes who have optimal levels of muscle glycogen and water have the energy necessary to work vigorously throughout the competitive event. Consequently, if you implement the above recommendations, you will be preventing your athletes from teetering on the weight control–energy management tightrope. At the same time, you will be complementing your athletes' physical training program.

Chapter 15
As the Caliper Turns

Athletes need not starve themselves and form poor nutritional habits. You can help your athletes avoid these pitfalls by taking the following measures:

- Determining athletes' optimal weight range based on individual body composition
- Applying the weight loss or weight gain guidelines prior to the start of the competitive season to enable athletes to obtain their optimum weight
- Encouraging athletes to maintain their optimum weight throughout the season by planning a nutritional diet and balancing their caloric consumption—particularly fat intake—with training and energy expenditure
- Incorporating strength and energy system training into your program
- Optimizing performance potentials by encouraging athletes to use the high-performance diet and pre-event meal suggestions

If you do all of these things, your athletes should be able to have a safe, successful, and enjoyable season. Furthermore, if you can get your athletes to use the weight control practices and dietary knowledge presented in this book, you will be helping them form valuable lifetime nutritional habits. They will learn to balance caloric consumption and expenditure, to restrict fat consumption and minimize salt intake, and to eat balanced nutritional meals.

But these outcomes will occur *only* if you are successful in getting your athletes to adopt sound nutritional and weight control practices. The use of the behavior modification strategies mentioned in chapter 11 and various motivational and reward systems may

help in this regard, but perhaps the most important tool can be found in the words of Edgar A. Guest.

> I'd rather see a sermon than hear one any day;
>
> I'd rather one should walk with me than merely tell the way.
>
> The eye's a better pupil and more willing than the ear,
>
> Fine counsel is confusing, but example's always clear;
>
> And the best of all the preachers are the men who live their creeds,
>
> For to see good put in action is what everybody needs.
>
> I soon can learn to do it if you'll let me see it done;
>
> I can watch your hands in action, but your tongue too fast may run.
>
> And the lecture you deliver may be very wise and true,
>
> But I'd rather get my lessons by observing what you do;
>
> For I might misunderstand you and the high advice you give,
>
> But there's no misunderstanding how you act and how you live.

From *Collected Verse of Edgar A. Guest*, p. 509. Copyright 1934 by Reilly & Lee Co. (now Contemporary Books). Reprinted with permission.

If you believe that optimal nutrition and body composition foster optimal performance, then respond to the Diet Habit Survey and turn the caliper on yourself to see if extra fat pounds are detracting from your own health and efficiency.

EATING HABITS

Complete the Diet Habit Survey in Appendix B. Are you at Phase III? That is the goal for all Americans. The total number of calories will not be as high for a coach who is not in an intensive training program, but the same low-fat diet that is optimal for the competing athlete is also optimal for health-related fitness. If you have not quite made it to Phase III, you and your athletes together can explore ways to minimize fat intake and seek out complex carbohydrates. If you are already at the Phase III level, you should have lots of practical tips to share with your athletes.

BODY COMPOSITION

Have a fellow coach take your skinfolds. Because you are a mature adult, you will use a different set of skinfolds and a nomogram (a special chart) to determine your percent fat. The specific directions for these skinfolds follow, but before you read this information, remember that the accuracy of these measurements depends upon locating the precise site for the skinfold and using the calipers correctly. Review chapter 2 for the instructions on calipers use before you begin.

Skinfolds for Women

The sites for taking skinfolds for body fat estimation of women include the triceps, suprailium, and thigh. All of these measurements are to be taken on the right side. The triceps skinfold is taken over the triceps muscle at the point exactly halfway between the elbow and the shoulder as presented in chapter 2. The suprailiac skinfold is taken by measuring the thickness of the diagonal fold of skin and fat just above the hipbone as illustrated in Figure 15.1. The site for the thigh skinfold is located by having the individual put her weight on the left leg and assume a stance with the right knee slightly flexed. A vertical fold in the front of the thigh, halfway between the hip and knee joints, is then taken (see Figure 15.2).

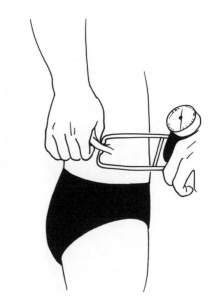

Figure 15.1. For adult females, take a suprailiac skinfold.

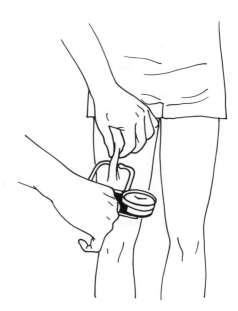

Figure 15.2. A thigh skinfold is also used in determining percent body fat in both women and men.

Skinfolds for Men

The skinfold sites for estimating percent fat for males are the chest, abdomen, and thigh. The chest skinfold site is over the outside or lateral border of the pectoralis major muscle. This site is depicted in Figure 15.3. The abdominal skinfold is a vertical fold located 1/2 to 1 inch to the right of the navel (Figure 15.4). The

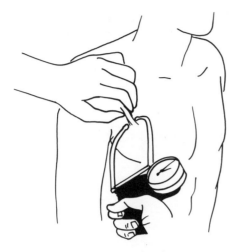

Figure 15.3. A chest skinfold is required to determine body fat in adult males.

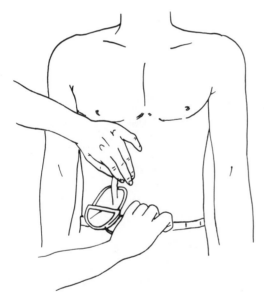

Figure 15.4. A skinfold taken near the navel is the final skinfold necessary for adult males.

thigh skinfold site is the same as that used for women and was described in the previous paragraph.

Determining Body Composition

Record three measurements for each of the three appropriate locations and calculate the average for each skinfold. Note your results on the form on page 144. Now total the three skinfold averages.

Locate the sum of the skinfold averages on the "Sum of Three Skinfolds" line on the right side of the nomogram in Figure 15.5 on page 145. Remember that a different set of skinfolds are used for males and females.

The other piece of information necessary to use the nomogram is the individual's age. Mark the appropriate age on the "Age in Years" line on the left side of the nomogram. Now use a pencil and a ruler or other straight-edge to connect the age and sum of three skinfold values. The percent fat value is the value at which the nomogram and your pencil line intersect. Be sure to look at the percent body fat line for the correct sex.

DETERMINING DESIRED BODY WEIGHT

To determine your optimal body weight, follow the same procedures that were presented in chapter 2:

$$\text{Optimal weight} = \frac{\text{Fat-free weight}}{100\% - \text{desired } \% \text{ fat}}$$

The desired percent fat range for nonathlete adults is 16% to 19% for males and 20% to 25% for females. These values are higher than those given for athletes because the average person is not trying to achieve maximal efficiency as an athlete is.

PUTTING IT ALL TOGETHER

Once you have determined your body composition, if you find that it is not in the desired range, follow recommendations in this book to begin taking off fat pounds. This action is a very powerful way to say, "I believe that optimal weight is important and I will follow a sound weight control program to lose fat weight." If you decide to take no action to reduce your own fat weight, there is no reason for your athletes to believe that optimal weight control is important for their performance or health reasons.

Coaches who always appear with a can of soda pop in one hand and a candy bar, chips, or other high-fat food in the other will have a great deal of difficulty convincing their athletes of the merits of avoiding junk foods and focusing on complex carbohydrates. Similarly, coaches who skip breakfast and lunch may experience a depressed blood glucose level and

Body Composition Prediction for Adults

Name _____ Date _____

Body weight _____ lb Sex _____

Ideal percent fat _____ Predicted percent fat _____

Fat-free weight (FFW) _____ lb Optimal body weight _____ lb

Skinfolds—Females

	#1	#2	#3	Average
Triceps	_____ mm	_____ mm	_____ mm =	_____ mm
Suprailiac	_____ mm	_____ mm	_____ mm =	_____ mm
Thigh	_____ mm	_____ mm	_____ mm =	_____ mm
			Sum of skinfolds =	_____ mm

Skinfolds—Males

	#1	#2	#3	Average
Chest	_____ mm	_____ mm	_____ mm =	_____ mm
Abdominal	_____ mm	_____ mm	_____ mm =	_____ mm
Thigh	_____ mm	_____ mm	_____ mm =	_____ mm
			Sum of skinfolds =	_____ mm

Desired weight

1. FFW = body weight − (% fat × body weight)

   FFW = _____ lb − (_____ × _____ lb)

   _____ lb = _____ lb − (_____ lb)

2. Optimal weight = $\dfrac{\text{FFW}}{(100\% - \text{desired } \% \text{ fat})}$

   Optimal weight = _____

   _____ lb = _____ lb

   _____ lb = _____

will likely find themselves in a foul mood by the time practice rolls around. Coaches like this simply cannot be sensitive to the individual needs of athletes and concentrate on running efficient and productive practice sessions. Don't allow yourself to fall into this situation.

SUMMARY AND RECOMMENDATIONS

Weight control is important for effective and efficient performance. It is true that lean individuals have fewer health problems than do obese individuals. So, preach nutrition and

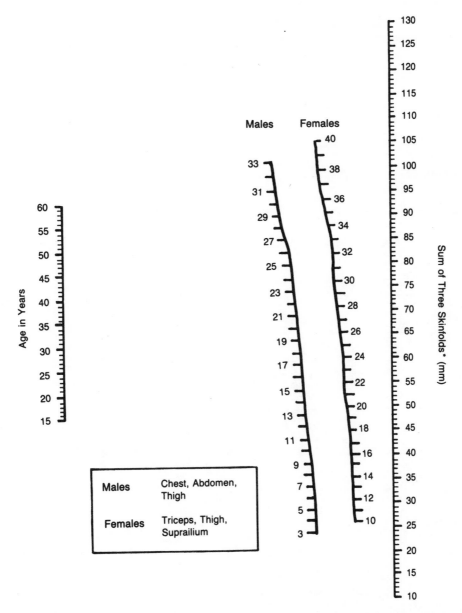

Figure 15.5. This nomogram can be used to estimate percent body fat for adult males and females based on age and the sum of three skinfold measurements. From "A Nomogram for the Estimate of Percent Body Fat from Generalized Equations" by W.B. Baun, M.R. Baun, and P.B. Raven, 1981, *Research Quarterly for Exercise and Sport*, **52**(3), p. 382. Copyright 1981 by the American Alliance for Health, Physical Education, Recreation and Dance. Reprinted by permission.

weight control—and practice what you preach! To do this you must take the following steps:

1. Assess your own personal body composition, and if your percent fat is not in the desired range, implement a fat control program.
2. Complete the Diet Habit Survey. If you are not at the Phase III level, begin to alter your dietary habits. Start gradually by selecting food choices with lower fat content. Rereading chapters 11 and 14 should provide you with some specific ways to decrease fat and substitute carbohydrate for fat.

Adopting a low-fat, high-carbohydrate diet will help you with fat control, provide you with more energy, and give you a great deal of insight to help you guide your athletes. Don't miss this opportunity to help them and yourself too.

Appendix A
Using the Adipometer

Many of the same instructions presented in chapter 2 on using the skinfold caliper apply to using the Adipometer skin caliper available from Ross Laboratories. The skinfolds are taken on the right side of the body. Use considerable care in locating the precise site for the measurement. Once you have located the correct site, firmly grasp the skin between the left thumb (right if you're left-handed) and forefinger and lift up the skin with its underlying fat tissue. Now, take the caliper in hand and place the "jaws" on either side of the skinfold. Place your thumb (index finger if you're left-handed) on the caliper's "trigger lever," which is marked "PRESS." An expensive and accurate caliper will have a built-in spring that exerts a constant tension on the jaws as they close on the skinfold. Because the Adipometer has no such spring, you must apply the tension by pressing the caliper together until the short black line on the trigger lever is aligned with the short black line (marked "ALIGN") on the main arm.

When these two lines are aligned, find the indicator line and read the measurement to the nearest millimeter. Release the tension and remove the caliper. Repeat this procedure three times for each skinfold site and record the values. Remember that these values may be somewhat less accurate than those taken with the more expensive caliper, but practice and good judgment will make the Adipometer a useful tool in your athletes' weight control program.

Appendix B
The Diet Habit Survey

Name _____

Date _____

The Diet Habit Survey
(A Quiz to Determine Your Need for Change)

This quiz was designed to enable you to evaluate your current eating habits and to compare them with the goals of the New American Diet. By taking this quiz now you will get some idea of what you need to do in order to achieve this way of eating. And by taking this same quiz at various times later on, you will be able to gauge your progress. Most of you, eating typical Western world fare, will not score particularly well at the outset. That is to be expected. This quiz will help you identify those areas in which you need work. If you fall far short of the goals, do not panic. Many of you have spent most of your lives getting into your current eating habits; do not expect to change them overnight. Slow, steady change is the path to permanent change.

Directions: For each question in each category, circle the numbers to the left of the answers that best describe your eating habits during the past month. The number at the left of each possible answer is the point score. Put that number in the blank space after each question. If you checked more than one answer for a question, put the average of the circled answers in the blank space (unless otherwise indicated). For example, with respect to question 5 under "Meat, Fish, and Poultry," if you checked bacon, sausage, etc., and also checked turkey ham, your score is $(1 + 3) \div 2 = 2$.

Compare your scores with goal scores at the end of the questionnaire.

Meat, Fish, and Poultry

For each question, circle as many numbers as apply and average them to get your score.

1. Which type of ground beef do you usually eat?
   - _1_ Regular hamburger (30% fat)
   - _2_ Lean ground beef (25% fat)
   - _3_ Extra lean/ground chuck (20% fat)
   - _4_ Super lean/ground round (15% fat)
   - _5_ Ground sirloin (10% fat) or eat no ground beef
   - ____ Score

Note. This appendix is from *The New American Diet* (pp. 41-51) by S.L. Connor and W.E. Connor, 1986, New York: Simon & Schuster. Copyright 1986 by Sonja L. Connor, M.S., R.D. and William E. Connor, M.D. Reprinted by permission of Simon and Schuster, Inc.

2. Which best describes your typical lunch?

__1__ Cheeseburger, typical cheeses, egg dishes (egg salad, quiche, etc.)

__2__ Sandwiches (lunch meat, hot dog, hamburger, fried fish, etc.) <u>or</u>, entree of meat or chicken (plain or fried)

__3__ Tuna sandwich, fish entree (not fried), entree with small bits of chicken or meat in a soup or casserole

__4__ Peanut butter sandwich

__5__ Salad, yogurt, cottage cheese, vegetarian dishes (without high-fat cheeses or egg yolk)

_____ Score

3. Which of these reflect your choices for the entree at your main meal?

__1__ Cheese (Cheddar, Jack, etc.), eggs, liver, heart, or brains <u>once a week or more</u>

__2__ Beef, lamb, pork, or ham <u>once a week or more</u>

__3__ Very lean red meat (top round or flank steak), veal, venison, or elk <u>once a week or more</u>

__4__ Chicken, turkey, rabbit, crab, lobster, or shrimp <u>twice a week or more</u>

__5__ Fish, scallops, oysters, clams, or meatless dishes containing no egg yolk or high-fat cheese <u>twice a week or more</u>

_____ Score

4. Estimate the number of ounces of meat, cheese, fish, and poultry you eat in a typical day. Include all meals and snacks.
   To guide you in your estimate:

   Meat in most sandwiches = 2-3 oz
   Chicken thigh   = 2-3 oz
   4 strips bacon   = 1 oz
   1/2 chicken breast   = 3 oz
   Small burger patty   = 3 oz
   Average T-bone steak   = 8 oz
   1 slice cheese   = 1 oz
   1-inch cube cheese   = 1 oz

   __1__ 11 or more ounces <u>a day</u>

   __2__ 9 to 10 ounces <u>a day</u>

   __3__ 6 to 8 ounces <u>a day</u>

   __4__ 4 to 5 ounces <u>a day</u>

   __5__ Not more than 1 ounce of cheese, 3 ounces of red meat, poultry, shrimp, crab, lobster or not more than 6 ounces of fish, clams, oysters, scallops <u>a day</u>

   _____ Score

5. Which of these have you eaten in the past month?

   _1_ Bacon, sausage, bologna; and other lunch meats, pepperoni; beef or pork wieners

   _2_ Canadian bacon, turkey wieners

   _3_ Turkey ham and other poultry lunch meats

   _4_ Soy products (breakfast links)

   _5_ None

   ____ Score

Total score _____ (Add all of the above scores in this category.)

Dairy Products and Eggs

For each question, circle as many numbers as apply and average them to get your score.

6. Which kind of milk do you usually use for drinking or cooking?

   _1_ Whole milk

   _2_ 2% milk

   _4_ 1% milk

   _5_ Skim milk, nonfat dry milk, or none

   ____ Score

7. Which toppings do you use?

   _1_ Sour cream (real or imitation including IMO*), whipped cream

   _3_ Nondairy toppings (Cool Whip or Dream Whip)

   _4_ Regular cottage cheese, whole milk yogurt

   _5_ Low-fat cottage cheese, low-fat yogurt, or none

   ____ Score

8. Which frozen desserts are you most likely to eat at least once a month?

   _1_ Ice cream

   _3_ Ice milk, most soft ice cream, Tofutti, frozen yogurt (cream added)

   _4_ Sherbet, low-fat frozen yogurt

   _5_ Sorbets, ices, popsicles, or none

   ____ Score

---

*Certain products are listed to provide examples of food items available. There may be other products of similar composition with different trade names.

9. Which kind of cheese do you use for snacks or sandwiches?

   __1__ Cheddar, Swiss, Jack, Brie, feta, American, cream cheese, regular cheese slices, or cheese spreads

   __2__ Part-skim mozzarella, Lappi, light cream cheese or Neufchatel, part-skim Cheddar (Kraft Light, Green River, Olympia's Low Fat, or Heidi Ann Low-Fat Ched-Style Cheese)

   __4__ Low-cholesterol "filled" cheese (Scandic Mini Chol [Swedish low cholesterol], Hickory Farms Lyte, or Cheezola)

   __5__ Very-low-fat processed cheese (Dorman's Light, Reduced Calories Laughing Cow, Weight Watchers, or the Lite-line series of cheeses), or no cheese

   _____ Score

10. Which kind of cheese do you use in cooking (casseroles, vegetables, etc.)?

   __1__ Cheddar, Swiss, Jack, Brie, feta, American, cream cheese, processed cheese (note: most restaurants use these)

   __3__ Part-skim mozzarella, Lappi, light cream cheese, part-skim Cheddar (Green River, Olympia's Low Fat, Kraft Light, or Heidi Ann Low-fat Ched-Style Cheese)

   __4__ Low-cholesterol "filled" cheese (Scandic Mini Chol [Swedish low cholesterol], Hickory Farms Lyte, or Cheezola)

   __5__ Very-low-fat processed cheese (Dorman's Light, Reduced Calories Laughing Cow, Weight Watchers, or the Lite-line series of cheeses), or no cheese

   _____ Score

11. Check the type and number of "visible" eggs you eat.

   __1__ Six or more whole eggs <u>a week</u>

   __2__ Three to five whole eggs <u>a week</u>

   __3__ One to two whole eggs <u>a week</u>

   __4__ One whole egg <u>a month</u>

   __5__ Egg white, egg substitute such as Egg Beaters, Scramblers, Second Nature, or none

   _____ Score

12. Check the type of eggs usually used in food prepared at home or bought in grocery stores (baked goods, such as cakes and cookies, potato and pasta salads, pancakes, etc.)

   __1__ Whole eggs or mixes containing whole eggs (complete pancake mix, slice-and-bake cookies, etc.)

   __3__ Combination of egg white, egg substitute, and whole egg

   __5__ Egg white, egg substitute, or none

   _____ Score

Total score _____ (Add all of the above scores in this category.)

Fats and Oils

For each question, circle as many numbers as apply and average them to get your score.

13. Which kinds of fat are used most often to cook your food (vegetables, meats, etc.)?

    __1__ Butter, shortening (all brands except Crisco or Food Club) or lard, bacon grease, chicken fat, or eat in restaurants at least 4 times a week

    __3__ Soft shortening (Crisco or Food Club) or inexpensive stick margarine (remains hard at room temperature)

    __4__ Tub or soft-stick margarine, vegetable oil

    __5__ None or use nonstick pan or spray

    _____ Score

14. Which best describes your daily use of these "visible" fats?

    (One serving = 1 teaspoon margarine, butter, oil, mayonnaise, Miracle Whip

    OR

    One serving = 2 teaspoons imitation or light mayonnaise, salad dressing, peanut butter, diet margarine)

    Typical Amounts:

On toast	= 2 tsp margarine, butter
On sandwiches	= 3 tsp mayonnaise
	= 6 tsp peanut butter
	= 2 tsp margarine, butter
On salads	= 12 tsp salad dressings
On potatoes or vegetables	= 3 tsp margarine

    __1__ 10 servings or more

    __2__ 8 to 9 servings

    __3__ 6 to 7 servings

    __4__ 4 to 5 servings

    __5__ 3 servings or less

    _____ Score

15. How often do you eat potato chips, corn or tortilla chips, fried chicken, fish sticks, french fries, doughnuts, other fried foods, croissants, or Danish pastries?

    __1__ 2 or more times a day

    __2__ One a day

    __3__ 2 to 4 times a week

    __4__ Once a week

    __5__ Less than twice a month

    _____ Score

16. Which best describes the amount of margarine, peanut butter, mayonnaise, or cream cheese that you put on breads, muffins, bagels, etc.?

    __1__ Average (1 teaspoon or more per serving)

    __2__ Lightly spread (can see through it)

    __4__ "Scrape" (can barely see it)

    __5__ None

    _____ Score

17. Which kind of salad dressings do you use?

    __1__ Real mayonnaise, Roquefort, blue cheese, Thousand Island, 3/4 oil and 1/4 vine-
    gar, ranch salad dressing made with sour cream, IMO, or mayonnaise

    __2__ Miracle Whip

    __3__ Imitation or light mayonnaise, Miracle Whip Light, Italian, ranch salad dressing
    made with buttermilk and sour cream, IMO, or mayonnaise

    __4__ French, garlic, 1/3 oil and 2/3 vinegar, ranch salad dressing made with butter-
    milk and imitation or light mayonnaise or Miracle Whip Light

    __5__ Low-calorie dressing, vinegar, lemon juice, ranch salad dressing made with but-
    termilk and low-fat yogurt, or use no salad dressing

    _____ Score

Total score _____ (Add all of the above scores in this category.)

Grains, Beans, Fruits, and Vegetables

For this part of the quiz, give yourself 5 points for each serving of the following foods you
eat each <u>day</u> or <u>week</u> as specified.

18. Give yourself 5 points for each piece of fruit or each cup of fruit juice consumed <u>a day</u>
    (not "fruit-flavored" drinks).

    _____ Score

19. Give yourself 5 points for each cup of vegetables eaten <u>a day</u> (tossed salad, cooked vege-
    tables, etc.).

    _____ Score

20. Give yourself 5 points for each cup of legumes eaten <u>a week</u> (refried beans, split peas,
    navy beans, lentils, chili, etc.)

    _____ Score

21. Give yourself 5 points for each small baked potato, 1/2 cup of cooked potatoes, macaroni,
    or other pasta, and 1/3 cup of rice or any other grain eaten <u>a day</u>

    _____ Score

22. Give yourself 5 points for each of the following eaten <u>a day</u>:

    1 slice bread   1/2 cup cooked cereal
    1 dinner or hard roll   1 cup ready-to-eat cereal
    1/2 hamburger bun   One 4-inch pancake
    1/2 bagel or English muffin   3 cups popcorn (no fat added)
    5 low-fat crackers   1 average muffin
    One 6-inch tortilla

    _____ Score

23. It is important to eat from each food group regularly. Therefore, <u>subtract</u> 5 points for each question 18 through 22 that received a zero score.

_____ Total subtracted

Total score _____ (Add scores for 18 through 22 above and <u>subtract</u> the score for 23 to get total score.)

Sweets, Snacks, and Beverages

For each question, circle as many numbers as apply and average them to get your score.

24. How often do you eat dessert or baked goods (sweet rolls, doughnuts, cookies, cakes, etc.)?
    <u>1</u> Three or more times <u>a day</u>
    <u>2</u> Two times <u>a day</u>
    <u>3</u> Once <u>a day</u>
    <u>4</u> 4 to 6 times <u>a week</u>

    _____ Score

25. Which of the following reflects your habits regarding alcoholic beverages?
    1 drink = 12 ounces beer
    　　　　1-1/2 ounces whiskey, gin, rum, etc.
    　　　　4 ounces wine
    　　　　1 ounce liqueur

    <u>1</u> 1 or more drinks <u>a day</u>
    <u>2</u> 4 to 6 drinks <u>a week</u>
    <u>3</u> 3 drinks <u>a week</u>
    <u>4</u> 1 to 2 drinks <u>a week</u>
    <u>5</u> None or less than <u>one a week</u>

    _____ Score

26. Which of the following reflects your habits regarding sweetened soda pop?
    12 ounce can = 1-1/2 cups
    16-oz bottle = 2 cups
    32-oz bottle = 4 cups

    <u>1</u> 1 or more cups a day or 7 cups <u>a week</u>
    <u>2</u> 4 to 6 cups <u>a week</u>
    <u>3</u> 3 cups <u>a week</u>
    <u>4</u> 1 to 2 cups <u>a week</u>
    <u>5</u> None or less than one cup <u>a week</u>

    _____ Score

27. How much regular coffee do you drink?
    __1__ 6 or more cups <u>a day</u>
    __3__ 4 to 5 cups <u>a day</u>
    __4__ 1 to 3 cups <u>a day</u>
    __5__ None or less than 1 cup <u>a day</u>

    _____ Score

28. Which of the following are you most likely to select as a dessert choice?
    __1__ Croissants, pies, cheesecake, carrot cake
    __2__ Regular cakes, cupcakes, cookies
    __3__ Combination of regular and low-fat desserts
    __5__ Fruits, low-fat cookies (fig bars and gingersnaps), angel food cake, low-fat muffins, desserts from low-fat cookbooks, or none

    _____ Score

29. Which snack items are you most likely to eat in an average month?
    __1__ Chocolate
    __2__ Potato chips, corn or tortilla chips, nuts, party/snack crackers, doughnuts, french fries, peanut butter, cookies
    __4__ Lightly buttered popcorn (1 tsp for 3 cups), pretzels, low-fat crackers (soda, graham), "home"-baked corn chips, low-fat cookies (gingersnaps, fig bars)
    __5__ Fruit, vegetables, very low-fat snacks, or none

    _____ Score

Total score _____ (Add all of the above scores in this category.)

Salt

For each question, circle as many numbers as apply and average them to get your score.

30. Which type of "salt" do you normally use?
    __1__ Regular salt, sea salt, flavoring salts (garlic, onion, celery salt), regular soy sauce
    __3__ Combination or regular and reduced sodium salts
    __4__ Lite Salt, lower-sodium soy sauce, reduced-sodium flavoring salts
    __5__ Salt substitute (100% potassium chloride), or none

    _____ Score

31. How often do you add salt to your food at the table?
    __1__ Always
    __2__ Frequently
    __4__ Occasionally
    __5__ Never

    _____ Score

32. Which type of salt and how much do you use in cooking potatoes, rice, pasta, vegetables, meat, casseroles, and soups?

    __1__ Regular salt (typical amount) or eat in restaurants 4 or more times <u>a week</u>

    __2__ Regular salt (1/2 typical amount) or Lite Salt (typical amount)

    __4__ Lite Salt (1/2 typical amount)

    __5__ Salt substitute or no salt used

    _____ Score

33. Which type of cereals do you use?

    __1__ Typical dry cereals (sweetened or unsweetened) or cereals cooked with regular salt (typical amount)

    __3__ Combination of typical dry cereals and salt-free dry cereals (Shredded Wheat, Puffed Wheat, Puffed Rice) or cereals cooked with regular salt (1/2 typical amount) or Lite Salt (typical amount)

    __5__ Salt-free dry cereals or cereals cooked with salt substitute or without salt or do not eat cereal

    _____ Score

34. How often do you use typical canned, bottled, or packaged foods: salad dressings, ketchup, cured meats (lunch meat, ham, etc.), vegetables, soups (remember chicken broth), chili, entrees, and sauces?

    __1__ More than 15 times <u>a week</u> or eat in restaurant 4 or more times <u>a week</u>

    __2__ 10 to 14 times <u>a week</u>

    __3__ 6 to 9 times <u>a week</u>

    __5__ Never to 5 times <u>a week</u>

    _____ Score

Total score _____ (Add all of the above scores in this category.)

Food Choices in Restaurants

35. Give yourself 5 points for EACH choice you make when eating in restaurants.

    __5__ Order toast, muffins, cereal, pancakes, waffles for breakfast

    __5__ Do not order fried, poached or scrambled eggs, omelettes, souffles, custards, cream pies, etc.

    __5__ Order soup (not cream), salad or other meatless, cheeseless entrees for lunch

    __5__ When ordering pizza choose vegetarian with a thick crust

    __5__ At the salad bar, avoid cheese, eggs, bacon bits, and potato and macaroni salads

    __5__ Select no more than one high-fat item per meal—even on special occasions

    __5__ Order a fish, shellfish, chicken, or lean read meat entree (but not fried)

    __5__ Order entrees broiled, poached, or baked but not fried or with no cream, cheese, or butter sauce

_5_ Use no more than 2 pats of margarine on a large baked potato (no sour cream or bacon bits)

_5_ Order oil and vinegar or a low-calorie salad dressing instead of Roquefort, blue cheese, sour cream, Thousand Island salad dressings and request that the salad dressing be served on the side (and use a very small amount)

_5_ Put garbanzo or kidney beans on salad at the salad bar

_5_ Order fruit, sorbets, frozen yogurt, or skip dessert

_5_ Choose skim milk or water

_5_ Eat very low-fat meals the day before or the day after you eat out

_5_ Select restaurants that offer low-fat choices and order those choices

_____ Score (If you eat out less than once a month give yourself a score of 75 points)

Overall Eating Style

For each question, circle the number that applies. This is your score.

36. How often do you have low-fat, high-carbohydrate days?

_1_ Twice <u>a month or less</u>

_2_ Once <u>a week</u>

_3_ 2 to 3 day <u>a week</u>

_4_ 4 to 5 days <u>a week</u>

_5_ 6 to 7 days <u>a week</u>

_____ Score

37. How often are low-fat recipes used in your house? (A low-fat bread, dessert, side dish or salad recipe contains no more than 1 teaspoon of fat per serving or less than 1/4 cup fat per recipe for 12 servings.)

_1_ Once <u>a month or less</u>

_2_ 1 to 2 times <u>a week</u>

_3_ 3 to 4 times <u>a week</u>

_4_ 5 to 6 times <u>a week</u>

_5_ Every day

_____ Score

Total score _____ (Add the above scores in this category.)

Assessment of the Diet Habit Survey Scores for 2,000 Calories
Women/Children

Place your score for each category of questions in the appropriate blank space. Circle the scores for each category that are similar to your score. See in which categories you score closer to Phase III goals and in which categories you score far from the goals. The TOTAL SCORE will give you an idea of your overall eating behavior pattern. The nutrients listed below the total scores will give you a good estimate of your diet composition. Finally, there is space for you to list at least three ways you can change your eating habits toward the Phase III goals.

	Present American diet	The New American Diet Phase I	II	III	Your score
Meat, fish, and poultry	< 12	12-13	16-18	21-25	_____
Dairy products and eggs	< 23	23-26	29-32	31-35	_____
Fats and oils	< 14	14-16	19-21	22-25	_____
Grains, beans, fruits, and vegetables	< 45	45-62	67-80	85-102	_____
Sweets, snacks, and beverages	< 18	18	24-28	29-30	_____
Salt	< 14	14-16	20	24-25	_____
Restaurant choices	< 15	15-35	40-60	65-75	_____
Overall eating style	< 6	6	8	10	_____
Total	<147	147-192	223-267	287-327	

These total scores correspond to a diet with the following nutrient composition:

Cholesterol, mg/day	400	<300	<200	<100	_____
Saturated fat, % calories	14	10	8	5	_____
Fat, % calories	40	35	25	20	_____
Carbohydrate, % calories	45	50	60	65	_____
Protein, % calories	15	15	15	15	_____
Sodium, mg/day	>2,875	2,875	2,300	1,725	_____
Potassium, mg/day	<2,535	2,535	3,900	3,900	_____

Suggestions for changing eating habits toward Phase III:

Assessment of the Diet Habit Survey Scores for 2,800 Calories
Men/Teens

Place your score for each category of questions in the appropriate blank space. Circle the scores for each category that are similar to your score. See in which categories you score closer to Phase III goals and in which categories you score far from the goals. The TOTAL SCORE will give you an idea of your overall eating behavior pattern. The nutrients listed below the total scores will give you a good estimate of your diet composition. Finally, there is space for you to list at least three ways you can change your eating habits toward the Phase III goals.

	Present American diet	The New American Diet Phase I	II	III	Your score
Meat, fish, and poultry	< 11	11-12	15-17	20-24	_____
Dairy products and eggs	< 23	23-26	29-32	31-35	_____
Fats and oils	< 13	13-15	18-20	21-24	_____
Grains, beans, fruits, and vegetables	< 70	70-91	98-123	129-160	_____
Sweets, snacks, and beverages	< 18	18	24-28	29-30	_____
Salt	< 14	14-16	20	24-25	_____
Restaurant choices	< 15	15-35	40-60	65-75	_____
Overall eating style	< 6	6	8	10	_____
Total	<170	170-219	252-308	329-383	_____

These total scores correspond to a diet with the following nutrient composition:

Cholesterol, mg/day	500	<350	<220	<140	_____
Saturated fat, % calories	14	10	8	5	_____
Fat, % calories	40	35	25	20	_____
Carbohydrate, % calories	45	50	60	65	_____
Protein, % calories	15	15	15	15	_____
Sodium, mg/day	>4,025	4,025	3,220	2,415	_____
Potassium, mg/day	<3,549	3,549	5,460	5,460	_____

Suggestions for changing eating habits toward Phase III:

The Diet Habit Survey
Goal Scores for Individual Questions for 2,000 Calories
Women/Children

Question number	Present American diet	The New American Diet Phase I	II	III
1	<2	2-3	3-4	4-5
2	<2	2	3	4-5
3	<3	3	3-4	3-5
4	<3	3	4	5
5	<2	2	3	5
6	<4	4	4	5
7	<4	4	5	5
8	<3	3	4	4-5
9	<2	2	4-5	4-5
10	<3	3	3-4	3-5
11	<4	4-5	4-5	5
12	<3	3-5	5	5
13	<3	3-4	3-4	4-5
14	<3	3	4	5
15	<3	3	4	5
16	<2	2	4	4-5
17	<3	3-4	4-5	4-5
18	<10	10-11	12-13	14-16
19	<5	5-8	9-12	13-16
20	<3	3-7	8-10	11-15
21	<3	3-7	8-12	13-18
22	<24	24-29	30-33	34-37
23	−5	0	0	0
24	<3	3	4-5	5
25	<3	3	4	4-5
26	<3	3	4	4-5
27	<3	3	4	4-5
28	<3	3	3-5	5
29	<3	3	4-5	4-5
30	<3	3	4	4-5
31	<4	4	5	5
32	<2	2-4	5	5
33	<3	3	3	5
34	<2	2	3	5
35	<15	15-35	40-60	65-75
36	<3	3	4	5
37	<3	3	4	5

The Diet Habit Survey
Goal Scores for Individual Questions for 2,800 Calories
Men/Teens

Question number	Present American diet	The New American Diet Phase		
		I	II	III
1	<2	2-3	3-4	4-5
2	<2	2	3	4-5
3	<3	3	3-4	3-5
4	<2	2	3	4
5	<2	2	3	5
6	<4	4	4	5
7	<4	4	5	5
8	<3	3	4	4-5
9	<2	2	4-5	4-5
10	<3	3	3-4	3-5
11	<4	4-5	4-5	5
12	<3	3-5	5	5
13	<3	3-4	3-4	4-5
14	<2	2	3	4
15	<3	3	4	5
16	<2	2	4	4-5
17	<3	3-4	4-5	4-5
18	<15	15-18	19-21	22-25
19	<8	8-12	13-17	18-22
20	<10	10-15	16-19	20-25
21	<5	5-9	10-19	20-35
22	<32	32-37	40-47	49-53
23	−5	0	0	0
24	<3	3	4-5	5
25	<3	3	4	4-5
26	<3	3	4	4-5
27	<3	3	4	4-5
28	<3	3	3-5	5
29	<3	3	4-5	4-5
30	<3	3	4	4-5
31	<4	4	5	5
32	<2	2-4	5	5
33	<3	3	3	5
34	<2	2	3	5
35	<15	15-35	40-60	65-75
36	<3	3	4	5
37	<3	3	4	5

Appendix C
Carbohydrate Sources

Low-Fat Complex Carbohydrates

Sources with 30 grams of carbohydrate per serving:

Breads
Bagel—1 small
Bun—1 (hamburger or hot dog)
English muffin—1
Matzo—1

Miscellaneous
Burrito (bean)—1
Tostado (bean)—1

Sources with 15 grams of carbohydrate per serving:

Breads and cereals
Bread (all kinds)—1 slice
Breadstick—2
Roll, tortilla (corn or wheat)—1
Cooked cereals—1/2 cup
English muffin—1
Ready-to-eat cereals—3/4 to 1 cup
Pancake or waffle—1 (5″ × 1/2″)

Crackers and snacks
Animal crackers—10
Graham crackers—2
Kavali crackers—3
Popcorn (air-popped)—3 cups
Pretzels (3-1/8″ long & 1/2″ diameter)—25

Rye crackers—2 rectangles
Roman Meal crackers—4
Rice cakes—2
Oyster crackers—20
Puffed wheat cakes—2
Saltine crackers—6

Pasta and rice
Macaroni, noodles, spaghetti (cooked, plain, or with tomato sauce)—1/2 cup
Ravioli (spinach)—1/2 cup
Rice (brown, white)—1/4 cup
Rice-a-Roni (prepared without fat)—1/2 cup

Dried beans, peas, and lentils
Baked beans—1/4 cup
Beans (kidney, lima, navy, northern, with pork, red)—1/2 cup
Lentils—1/2 cup
Peas (black-eyed, green, split)—1/2 cup

Soup
Bean (all)—1/2 cup
Noodle soup—1 cup
Minestrone—1 cup

Vegetables
Corn—1 small ear or 1/2 cup
Potatoes—1 small, 1/2 cup, or approximately 1/2 cup mashed
Winter squash—1/2 cup
Yam or sweet potato—1/4 cup

Sources with 5 grams of carbohydrate per 1/2-cup serving:

Asparagus	Spinach
Bean sprouts	Turnip
Beets	Mushrooms
Broccoli	Okra
Brussels sprouts	Onion
Cabbage	Rhubarb
Cauliflower	Rutabaga
Celery	Sauerkraut
Cucumber	String beans
Eggplant	Summer squash
Green pepper	Tomatoes
Beet greens	Tomato juice
Chard greens	Vegetable juice
Dandelion greens	cocktail
Kale greens	Zucchini
Mustard greens	

Low-Fat Simple Carbohydrates—*Contain Sugars as the Carbohydrate Source*

Sources with 35-40 grams of carbohydrate per serving:

Chocolate milk (2%) or instant cocoa—1 cup
Frozen yogurt—1 cup
Fudgesicle or popsicle—1-1/2
Nonfat fruit yogurt—1 cup
Pudding made with skim milk—1/2 cup
Sherbet or fruit ices—1 cup

Sources with 20 grams of carbohydrate per servings:

Dried Fruit
Apple rings—5
Apricot halves—10
Dates—3
Figs—1
Peach halves—3
Pear halves—3
Raisins—1 ounce

Sources with 12 grams of carbohydrate per serving:

Milk (skim, Buttermilk, 1% fat)—1 cup
Nonfat yogurt (plain)—1 cup

Sources with 10 grams of carbohydrate per serving:

Fresh Fruit and Juices
Apple—1 small
Apple juice—1/3 cup
Applesauce (unsweetened)—1/2 cup
Apricots (fresh)—2 medium
Banana—1/2 small
Berries—
 • Blackberries—1/4 cup
 • Blueberries—1/2 cup
 • Raspberries—1/2 cup
 • Strawberries—3/4 cup
Cherries—10 large
Figs—1
Grapefruit—1/2
Grapes—12
Grapejuice—1/4 cup
Mango—1/2 small
Melon—
 • Cantaloupe—1/4 small
 • Honeydew—1/8 medium
 • Watermelon—1 cup
 • Nectarine—1 small
Orange—1 small
Orange juice—1/2 cup
Peach—1 medium
Pear—1 medium

Cookies, Candies, Bakery Foods, Sweet Drinks
Angel food cake—1 slice (30 grams)
Carbondated soda—12 ounces (30-40 grams)
Fig bars—1 (11 grams)
Fruit punch/Kool Aid—10 ounces (35-40 grams)
Ginger snaps—4 (20 grams)
Hard candy (peppermint, butterscotch, etc.)—1 piece (5 grams)
Jelly beans—9 (15 grams)
Licorice (red or black)—1 ounce (25 grams)

Medium-Fat Sources of Complex Carbohydrates—*25-40% Calories From Fat*

Sources with 15 grams of carbohydrate:

Breads and Bakery Foods
Biscuit—1

Cornbread—2 × 2 × 1
Gingerbread—2 × 2 × 1
Muffins—1
Pancake—1
Waffle—1
Wheat germ—1/4 cup

Crackers and Snacks
Round butter-type crackers—5
Triscuits—5
Wheat Thins—9
Wheatsworth crackers—4 small squares

Pasta Dishes
Lasagna (cheese)—1/2 cup
Macaroni and cheese—1/2 cup
Ravioli (cheese)—1/2 cup

Miscellaneous
Beef or cheese burrito, taco, or tostada—1
Pizza (vegetable or plain cheese)—1 slice

High-Fat Sources of Carbohydrates—
45-70% Calories From Fat

Sources with 15 grams of simple and complex carbohydrate:

Cereals, Vegetables, and Snacks
Cheese crackers or puffs—10

French fries—8
Granola-type cereal—1/3 cup
Potato or corn chips—1 ounce (15 chips)

Cookies and Bakery Foods, Sweets
Brownie—2 small
Butter or shortbread cookie—2
Cake with icing—1 small piece
Chocolate candy—1 ounce
Chocolate chip cookie—1
Danish pastry—1 small
Doughnut—1
Pie (fruit or cream)—1/2 small piece

Soups
Cream soups (all types)—1 cup

Miscellaneous
Pepperoni or sausage pizza—1 slice

Sources with *35-40 grams* of simple carbohydrate:

Chocolate whole milk—1 cup
Custard—1/2 cup
Eggnog—1 cup
Ice cream—1 cup
Malt or milkshake—1 cup
French-style yogurt—1 cup
Gelatin dessert—1 cup

References

Acheson, K.J., Flatt, J.P., & Jequier, E. (1982). Glycogen synthesis versus lipogenesis after a 500 gram carbohydrate meal in man. *Metabolism*, **31**(12), 1234-1240.

Acheson, K.J., Schutz, Y., Bessard, T., Ravussin, E., & Jequier, E. (1984). Nutritional influences on lipogenesis and thermogenesis after a carbohydrate meal. *American Journal of Physiology*, **246**, E62-E70.

Alexiou, D., Anagnostopoulos, A., & Papadatos, C. (1979). Total free amino acids, ammonia and protein in the sweat of children. *American Journal of Clinical Nutrition*, **32**, 750-752.

Allen, L.H. (1982). Calcium bioavailability and absorption: A review. *American Journal of Clinical Nutrition*, **35**, 783-808.

Allen, L.H. (1984). Calcium absorption and requirements during the life span. *Nutrition News*, **47**(1), 1-3.

American Academy of Pediatrics. (1982). Climatic heat stress and the exercising child. *Pediatrics*, **69**, 808-809.

American Academy of Pediatrics. (1983). Weight training and weight lifting information for the pediatrician. *The Physician and Sportsmedicine*, **11**(8), 157-161.

American College of Sports Medicine. (1976). Position stand on weight loss in wrestlers. *Medicine and Science in Sports*, **8**(2), xi-xiii.

American College of Sports Medicine (1984). *Position stand on the use of anabolic-androgenic steroids in sports*. Indianapolis: Author.

Anderson, R.A., Polansky, M.M., Bryden, N.A., & Guttman, H.N. (1986). Strenuous exercise may increase dietary needs for chromium and zinc. In F.I. Katch (Ed.), *Sport, health, and nutrition* (pp. 83-88). Champaign, IL: Human Kinetics.

Astrand, P.O., & Saltin, B. (1964). Plasma and red cell volume after prolonged severe exercise. *Journal of Applied Physiology*, **19**, 829-832.

Avioli, L.V. (1987). The calcium controversy and the recommended dietary allowance. In L.V. Avioli (Ed.), *The osteoporotic syndrome: Detection, prevention, and treatment* (2nd ed.) (pp. 57-66). Orlando: Grune & Stratton.

Bar-or, O., Dotan, R., Inbar, O., Rotshtein, A., & Zonder, H. (1980). Voluntary hypohydration in 10-12 year-old boys. *Journal of Applied Physiology*, **48**, 104-108.

Becque, D., Katch, V.L., & Moffat, R.J. (1986). Time course of skin-plus-fat compression in males and females. *Human Biology*, **58**(1), 33-42.

Belko, A.Z., Obarzanek, E., Kalkwarf, H.J., Rotter, M.A., Bogusz, S., Miller, D., & Haas, J.D. (1983). Effects of exercise on riboflavin requirements of young women. *American Journal of Clinical Nutrition*, **37**(4), 509-517.

Bergstrom, J., Hermansen, L., Hultman, E., & Saltin, B. (1967). Diet muscle glycogen, and physical performance. *Acta Physiologica Scandinavica*, **71**, 140-150.

Bergstrom, J., & Hultman, E. (1972). Nutrition for maximal sports performance. *Journal of the American Medical Association*, **221**(9), 999-1006.

Besset, A., Bonardet, A., Roundouin, G., Descomps, B., & Passouant, P. (1982). Increase in sleep related GH and Prl secretion after chronic arginine aspartate administration in man. *Acta Endocrinologica*, **99**, 18-23.

Blanchard, D. (1972, March). How Stanford beat the weight loss problem. *Scholastic Coach*, pp. 88-90.

Bock, W., Fox, E.L., & Bowers, R. (1967). The effects of acute dehydration upon cardiorespiratory endurance. *Journal of Sport Medicine*, **7**, 67-72.

Boileau, R.A., Lohman, T.G., & Slaughter,

M.H. (1985). Exercise and body composition of children and youth. *Scandinavian Journal of Sports Science*, **7**(1), 17-27.

Brin, M., & Bauernfeind, J.C. (1978). Vitamin needs of the elderly. *Postgraduate Medicine*, **63**(3), 155-163.

Brooks, G.A. (1987). Amino acid and protein metabolism during exercise and recovery. *Medicine and Science in Sports and Exercise*, **19**(5), S150-S156.

Cade, J. (1971). Changes in body fluid composition and volume during vigorous exercise by athletes. *Journal of Sports Medicine and Physical Fitness*, **11**, 172-177.

Cade, J., Spooner, G., Schlein, E., Pickering, M., & Dean, R. (1972). Effect of fluid, electrolyte, and glucose replacement during exercise on performance, body temperature, rate of sweat loss and compositional changes of extracellular fluid. *Journal of Sports Medicine and Physical Fitness*, **12**, 150-156.

Cann, C.E., Martin, M.C., Genant, H.K., & Jaffe, R.B. (1984). Decreased spinal mineral content in amenorrheic women. *Journal of the American Medical Association*, **251**, 626-629.

Claremont, A.D., Costill, D.L., Fink, W., & Van Handel, P. (1976). Heat tolerance following diuretic induced dehydration. *Medicine and Science in Sports*, **8**, 239-243.

Clark, N. (1985). Increasing dietary iron. *The Physician and Sportsmedicine*, **13**(1), 131-132.

Clements, D.B., & Sawchuk, L.L. (1984). Iron status and sports performance. *Sports Medicine, Adis Press*, **1**, 65-74.

Colgan, M. (1982). *Your personal vitamin profile*. New York: William Morrow.

Colgan, M. (1987). Human growth hormone. *Muscle and Fitness*, **49**(1), 74, 76, 242-245.

Connor, S.L., & Connor, W.E. (1986). *The new American diet*. New York: Simon & Schuster.

Consolazio, C., Matoush, L.O., Nelson, R.A., Harding, R.S., & Canaham, J.E. (1963). Excretion of sodium, potassium, magnesium, and iron in human sweat and the relation of each to balance and requirements. *Journal of Nutrition*, **79**, 407-415.

Convertino, V.A., Brook, P.J., Keil, L.C., Bernauer, E.M., & Greenleaf, J.E. (1980). Exercise training-induced hypervolemia: Role of plasma albumin, renin and vasopressin. *Journal of Applied Physiology*, **48**, 665-669.

Costill, D.L. (1972). Water and electrolytes. In W. Morgan (Ed.), *Ergogenic aids and muscular performance*. New York: Academic.

Costill, D.L., Bowers, R.W., Branam, G., & Sparks, K. (1971). Muscle glycogen utilization during prolonged exercise on successive days. *Journal of Applied Physiology*, **31**, 834-838.

Costill, D.L., Branam, G., Fink, W.J., & Nelson, R. (1976). Exercise induced sodium conservation: Changes in plasma renin and aldosterone. *Medicine and Science in Sports*. **8**, 209-213.

Costill, D.L., Cote, R., Miller, E., Miller, T., & Wynder, S. (1975). Water and electrolyte replacement during repeated days of work in the heat. *Aviation, Space and Environmental Medicine*, **46**, 795-800.

Costill, D.L., Dalsky, D.L., & Fink, W.J. (1978). effects of caffeine ingestion on metabolism and exercise performance. *Medicine and Science in Sports*, **10**, 155-158.

Costill, D.L., & Higdon, H. (1981, July). Fat chance. *The Runner*, pp. 62-67.

Costill, D.L., Jansson, E., Gollnick, P.D., & Saltin, B. (1974). Glycogen utilization in leg muscles of men during level and uphill running. *Acta Physiologica Scandinavica*, **91**, 475-481.

Coyle, E.F., Coggan, A.R., Hemmert, M.K., & Ivy, J.L. (1986). Muscle glycogen utilization during prolonged strenuous exercise when fed carbohydrate. *Journal of Applied Physiology*, **61**, 165-172.

Coyle, E., Costill, D.L., Fink, W.J., & Hoopes, D.G. (1978). Gastric emptying rates for selected athletic drinks. *Research Quarterly*, **49**, 119-124.

Crooks, M. (1975, April). Protein supplementation and weight gain. *Scholastic Coach*, pp. 62-65.

Despres, J.P., Bouchard, C., Savard, R., Tremblay, A., Marcotte, M., & Theriault, G. (1984). Level of physical fitness and adipocyte lipolysis in humans. *Journal of Applied Physiology*, **56**, 1157-1164.

Dohm, G.L., Tapscott, E.B., & Kasperek, G.J. (1987). Protein degradation during endurance exercise and recovery. *Medicine and Science in Sports and Exercise*, **19**(5), S166-S171.

Donahoe, C., Lin, D.H., Kirschenbaum, D.S.,

& Keesey, R. (1984). Metabolic consequences of dieting and exercise in the treatment of obesity. *Journal of Consulting and Clinical Psychology*, **52**(5), 827-836.

Dressendorfer, R.H., Wade, C.E., Keen, C.L., & Scatf, J.H. (1982). Plasma mineral levels in marathon runners during a 20-day road race. *The Physician and Sportsmedicine*, **8**(6), 97-100.

Drinkwater, B.L., Nilson, K., Chestnut, C.H., Bremner, W.J., Shainholtz, S., & Southworth, M.B. (1984). Bone mineral content of amenorrheic and eumenorrheic athletes. *New England Journal of Medicine*, **311**, 277-281.

Duda, M. (1985). Baseball players are leaner—but better? *The Physician and Sportsmedicine*, **13**(6), 38-39.

Dunn, K. (1981). Menstrual, diet problems found in ballet dancers. *The Physician and Sportsmedicine*, **9**(8), 21-22.

Durnin, J.V.G.A. (1978). Protein requirements and physical activity. In J. Parizkova & V.A. Rogozkin (Eds.), *Nutrition, physical fitness, and health* (pp. 53-60). Baltimore: University Press.

Early, R., & Carlson, B. (1969). Water soluble vitamin therapy on the delay of fatigue from physical activity in hot climatic conditions. *Internationale Zeitschrift fuer Angewandte Physiologie Einschliesslich Arbeitsphysiologie*, **27**, 43-50.

Eichner, E.R. (1986). The anemias of athletes. *The Physician and Sportsmedicine*, **14**(9), 122-130.

Feinstein, R.A., & Daniel, W.A. (1984). Anemia and 'anemia' in adolescents: Value in screening examinations for sports. *The Physician and Sportsmedicine*, **12**(1), 140-144.

Fink, W. (1982). Fluid intake for maximizing athletic performance. In W. Haskel, J. Scala, & J. Whittam (Eds.), *Nutrition and athletic performance* (pp. 52-63). Palo Alto: Bull.

Foster, C., Costill, D.L., & Fink, W.J. (1979). Effects of preexercise feedings on endurance performance. *Medicine and Science in Sports*, **11**, 1-5.

Fox, E.L., & Mathews, D.K. (1976). The physiological basis of physical education and athletics. Philadelphia: W.B. Saunders.

Frizzell, R.T., Lang, G.H., Lowance, D.C., & Lathan, S.R. (1986). Hyponatremia and ultramarathon running. *Journal of the American Medical Association*, **255**(6), 772-774.

Gardner, G.W., Edgerton, V.R., Senewiratne, B., Baranard, R.J., & Ohira, Y. (1977). Physical work capacity and metabolic stress in subjects with iron deficiency anemia. *American Journal of Clinical Nutrition*, **30**, 910-917.

Girandola, R.N. (1976). Body composition changes in women: Effect of high and low exercise intensity. *Archives of Physical Medicine and Rehabilitation*, **56**(6), 297-300.

Greenleaf, J., & Castle, B. (1971). Exercise temperature regulation in man during hypohydration and hyperhydration. *Journal of Applied Physiology*, **30**, 847-853.

Guyton, A.C. (1981). *Textbook of medical physiology*. Philadelphia: W.B. Saunders.

Hackman, E.M. (1985). Water works. *Action*, **8**(6), 1-2.

Hawkins, J.D. (1983). An analysis of selected skinfold measuring instruments. *Journal of Physical Education, Recreation and Dance*, **54**(1), 25-27.

Haymes, E.M. (1983). Proteins, vitamins, and iron. In M.H. Williams (Ed.), *Ergogenic aids in sport* (pp. 27-55). Champaign, IL: Human Kinetics.

Hazeyama, Y., & Sparks, H. (1979). A model of potassium ion efflux during exercise of skeletal muscle. *American Journal of Physiology*, **236**, R83-R90.

Heaney, R.P. (1987). Prevention of osteoporotic fracture in women. In L.V. Avioli (Ed.), *The osteoporotic syndrome: Detection, prevention, and treatment* (2nd ed.) (pp. 67-90), Orlando: Grune & Stratton.

Herbert, W.G. (1983). Water and electrolytes. In M.H. Williams (Ed.), *Ergogenic aids in sport* (pp. 56-98). Champaign, IL: Human Kinetics.

Hultman, E., & Bergstrom, J. (1967). Muscle glycogan synthesis in relation to diet studied in normal subjects. *Acta Scandinavica Medilogica*, **182**, 109-117.

Knochel, J. (1977). Potassium deficiency during training in the heat. *Annals of the New York Academy of Science*, **301**, 175-182.

Kobayashi, Y. (1974). Effect of vitamin E on aerobic work performance in man during acute exposure to hypoxic hypoxia. (Unpublished Doctoral dissertation, University of New Mexico).

Lamb, S.R., & Brodowicz, G.R. (1986). Optimal use of fluids of varying formulations to minimize exercise-induced disturbances in homeostasis. *Sports Medicine*, **3**, 247-251.

Lane, H., & Cerda, J. (1979). Potassium requirements and exercise. *American Corrective Therapy Journal*, **33**, 67-69.

Laritcheva, K.A., Yalovaya, N.I., Shubin, V.I., & Smirnov, P.V. (1978). Study of the energy expenditure and protein needs of top weight lifters. In J. Parizkova & V.A. Rogozkin (Eds.), *Nutrition, physical fitness, and health* (pp. 155-164). Baltimore: University Park.

Larsson, L. (1982). Physical training effects on muscle morphology in sedentary males at different ages. *Medicine and Science in Sports and Exercise*, **11**, 203-206.

LaVielle, G.A., & Romsos, D.R. (1974, November). Meal eating and obesity. *Nutrition Today*, pp. 4-9.

Lemon, P.W.R. (1987). Protein and exercise: Update 1987. *Medicine and Science in Sports and Exercise*, **19**(5), S179-S190.

Lohman, T.G. (1981). Skinfolds and body density and their relation to body fatness: A review. *Human Biology*, **53**, 181-225.

Lohman, T.G. (1986). Applicability of body composition techniques and constants for children and youths. *Exercise and sport science review*, **14**, 325-357.

Lohman, T.G. (1987). *Measuring body fat using skinfolds* [Videotape]. Champaign, IL: Human Kinetics.

Mann, G. (1977). Nutrition for athletes. *Journal of the American Medical Association*, **237**, 1076.

McLeod, W.D., Hunter, S.C., & Etchison, B. (1983). Performance measurement and percent body fat in the high school athlete. *American Journal of Sports Medicine*, **11**(6), 390-397.

Mitchell, J.W. (1977). Energy exchanges during exercise. In E.R. Nadel (Ed.), *Problems with temperature regulation during exercise* (pp. 11-26). New York: Academic.

Morrow, J.R., Fridye, T., & Monaghen, S.D. (1986). Generalizability of the AAHPERD Health Related Skinfold Test. *Research Quarterly for Exercise and Sport*, **57**, 187-195.

National Dairy Council (1984). *Calcium: A summary of current research for the health professional*. Rosemont, IL: National Dairy Council.

National Dairy Council. (1985). Nutrition and the immune response. *Dairy Council Digest*, **56**(2), 7-11.

National Research Council Committee on Dietary Allowances. (1974). *Recommended dietary allowances*. Washington, DC: National Academy of Sciences.

National Research Council Committee on Dietary Allowances. (1980). *Recommended dietary allowances*. Washington, DC: National Academy of Sciences.

Nilson, K.L. (1986). Injuries in female distance runners. In B.L. Drinkwater (Ed.), *Female endurance athletes* (pp. 149-161). Champaign, IL: Human Kinetics.

Nose, H., Mack, G., Shi, X., & Nadel, E. (1988). Role of osmolality and plasma volume during rehydration in humans. *Journal of Applied Physiology*, **65**, 325-331.

Pate, R.R. (1983). Sports anemia: A review of the current research literature. *The Physician and Sportsmedicine*, **11**(2), 115-126.

Pate, R.R., Maguire, M., & Van Wyk, J. (1979). Dietary iron supplementation in women athletes. *The Physician and Sportsmedicine*, **7**(9), 81-86.

Pernow, B., & Saltin, B. (1971). Availability of substrates and capacity for prolonged heavy exercise in man. *Journal of Applied Physiology*, **31**, 412-422.

Pike, R.L., & Brown, M.L. (1975). *Nutrition: An integrated approach*. New York: John Wiley & Sons.

Plowman, S.A., & McSwegin, P.C. (1981). The effects of iron supplementation on female cross country runners. *Journal of Sports Medicine and Physical Fitness*, **21**, 407-416.

Povlou, K.N., Steffee, W.P., Lerman, R.H., & Burrows, B.A. (1985). Effects of dieting and exercise on lean body mass, oxygen uptake, and strength. *Medicine and Science in Sports and Exercise*, **17**(4), 466-471.

Puhl, J.L., Van Handel, P.J., Williams, L.L., Bradley, P.W., & Harms, S.J. (1985). Iron status and training. In N.K. Butts, T.T. Gushiken, & B. Zarins (Eds.), *The elite athlete* (pp. 209-236). Champaign, IL: Life Enhancement Publications.

Rasch, P., & Pierson, W. (1962). Protein dietary supplementation on muscular strength and hypertrophy. *American Journal of Clinical Nutrition*, **11**, 530-532.

Roche, A.F., Abdel-Malek, A.K., & Mukherjee, D. (1985). New approaches to clinical assessment of adipose tissue. In A.F. Roche (Ed.), *Body composition assessments in youth and adults: Report of the Sixth Ross Conference on Medical Research* (pp. 14-19). Columbus, OH: Ross Laboratories.

Rose, K. (1975). Warning for millions: Intense exercise can deplete potassium. *The Physician and Sportsmedicine*, **3**(5), 67.

Rose, L., Carroll, D.R., Lowe, S.L., Peterson, E.W., & Cooper, K.H. (1970). Serum electrolyte changes after marathon running. *Journal of Applied Physiology*, **29**, 449-451.

Rossander, L., Hallberg, L., & Bjorn-Rasmussen, E. (1979). Absorption of iron from breakfast cereals. *American Journal of Clinical Nutrition*, **32**(12), 2484-2489.

Rudman, D., & Williams, P.J. (1983). Megadose vitamins: Use and Misuse. *New England Journal of Medicine*, **309**, 488-489.

Scheur, J., & Tipton, C.M. (1977). Cardiovascular adaptations to physical training. *Annual Review of Physiology*, **39**, 221-251.

Segal, K., & Gutin, B. (1983). Thermic effect of food and exercise in lean and obese women. *Metabolism*, **32**(6), 581-589.

Sims, D. (1970, December). An evaluation of liquid food supplements. *Scholastic Coach*, 28-29.

Sinning, W.E., Dolny, D.G., Little, K.D., Cunningham, L.M., Racaniello, A., & Siconolfi, S.F. (1985). Validity of "generalized" equations for body composition analysis in male athletes. *Medicine and Science in Sports and Exercise*, **17**, 124-130.

Smith, N. (1978). *Food for sport*. Palo Alto: Bull.

Steenkamp, I., Fuller, C., Graves, J., Noakes, T.D., & Jacobs, P. (1986). Marathon running fails to influence RBC survival rates in iron-replete women. *The Physician and Sportsmedicine*, **14**(5), 89-95.

Stewart, J.C., Ahlquist, D.A., McGill, D.B., Ilstrup, D.M., Schwartz, S., & Owen, R.A. (1984). Gastrointestinal blood loss and anemia in runners. *Annals of Internal Medicine*, **100**, 843-845.

Tanner, J.M., Huges, P.C.R., Whitehouse, R.H., & Carter, B.S. (1977). Relative importance of growth hormone and sex steroids for the growth at puberty of trunk length, limb length, and muscle width in growth hormone-deficient children. *Journal of Pediatrics*, **89**(6), 1000-1008.

Tanner, J.M., & Whitehouse, R.H. (1967). The effect of human growth hormone on subcutaneous fat thickness in hypophysectotrophic and panhypopituitary dwarfs. *Journal of Endocrinology*, **39**, 263-275.

Tremblay, A., Boilard, F., Breton, M., Bessette, H., & Roberge, A.G. (1984). The effects of a riboflavin supplementation on the nutritional status and performance of elite swimmers. *Nutrition Research*, **4**, 201-208.

U.S. Department of Health, Education, and Welfare. (1972). *Ten-state nutrition survey, 1968-1970* (Department of Health, Education, and Welfare Publication No. [HSM] 72-8133). Washington, DC: U.S. Government Printing Office.

U.S. Department of Health, Education, and Welfare. (1974). *Preliminary findings of the first health and nutrition examination survey (HANES I), United States, 1971-72: Dietary intake and biochemical findings* (Department of Health, Education, and Welfare Publication No. [HRH] 74-1219-1). Washington, DC: U.S. Government Printing Office.

Van Itallie, T., Sinisterra, L., & Stare, F. (1960). Nutrition and athletic performance. In W. Johnson (Ed.), *Science and medicine of exercise and sports* (pp. 285-300). New York: Harper.

Verde, T., Shephard, R.J., Corey, P., & Moore, R. (1982). Sweat composition in exercise and in heat. *Journal of Applied Physiology*, **53**, 1540-1545.

Wheeler, K.B., & Banwell, J.G. (1986). Intestinal and electrolyte flux of glucose-polymer electrolyte solutions. *Medicine and Science in Sports and Exercise*, **18**, 436-439.

White, A., Handler, P., & Smith, E. (1973). *Principles of biochemistry*. New York: McGraw-Hill.

Whitney, E.N., & Hamilton, E.M.N. (1981). *Understanding nutrition*. New York: West.

Wilkerson, J.E., Horvath, S.M., Gutin, B., Molnar, S., & Diaz, F.J. (1982). Plasma electrolyte content and concentration during treadmill exercise in humans. *Journal of Applied Physiology*, **53**, 1529-1539.

Williams, M.H. (1985). *Nutritional aspects of human physical and athletic perfor-*

mance. Springfield, IL: Charles C Thomas.

Wilmore, J.H., & Haskell, W.L. (1972). Body composition and endurance capacity of professional football players. *Journal of Applied Physiology*, **33**(5), 564-567.

Wintrobe, M.W. (1981). *Clinical hematology* (8th ed.). Philadelphia: Lea & Febiger.

Yoshimura, H. (1970). Anemia during physical training (sports anemia). *Nutrition Reviews*, **28**, 251-253.

Index

About the Authors

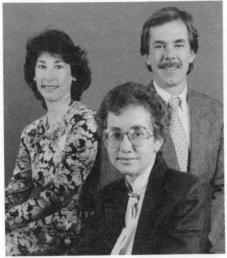

Joan Benson   **Stephen Johnson**
Patricia Eisenman

Patricia A. Eisenman, PhD, is the associate dean of the College of Health and executive director of the PEAK (Performance Enhancement through Applied Knowledge) Academy at the University of Utah. Dr. Eisenman has conducted extensive research in the areas of body composition and nutrition supplementation. She has also experienced success in coaching and attributes that success to her application and integration of the sport sciences. In conjunction with her professional responsibilities, Dr. Eisenman is a member of the American Alliance for Health, Physical Education, Recreation and Dance (AAHPERD) and the American College of Sports Medicine (ACSM), and a founder of the Utah Fitness Instructor's Association.

Stephen C. Johnson, PhD, is an assistant professor of exercise and sport science, adjunct professor of the Division of Foods and Nutrition, and director of the Human Performance Laboratory at the University of Utah. Dr. Johnson is a member of the Sports Medicine Council of the United States Ski Team as director of physiology. In addition to being a member of AAHPERD and ACSM, Dr. Johnson is a past recipient of the Utah Governor's Council for Health and Fitness award for his outstanding contribution to fitness.

Joan E. Benson, MS, RD, is an adjunct instructor of nutrition at the University of Utah and a nutrition consultant for the Center for Sports Medicine in San Francisco, where she teaches a course on nutrition and eating disorders. Ms. Benson has also published many articles and papers on the nutritional needs of athletes. She is a member of the American Dietetic Association and Sports and Cardiovascular Nutritionists (SCAN).